DATE DUE

Contributions to Psychology and Medicine

Contributions to Psychology and Medicine

Stephen Bochner

The Psychology
of the Dentist-Patient
Relationship

Springer-Verlag
New York Berlin Heidelberg
London Paris Tokyo

1988

Stephen Bochner
School of Psychology
University of New South Wales
Kensington, New South Wales 2033
Australia

Advisor
J. Richard Eiser
Department of Psychology
University of Exeter
Exeter EX4 4QG
England

Library of Congress Cataloging-in-Publication Data
Bochner, Stephen.
  The psychology of the dentist-patient relationship/Stephen
Bochner.
     p.   cm.—(Contributions to psychology and medicine)
  Bibliography: p.
  Includes indexes.
  ISBN 0-387-96642-0
  1. Dentistry—Psychological aspects.   2. Dentist and patient.
I. Title.   II. Series.
RK53.B66   1988
617.6'023—dc19   87-33098

Typeset by Asco Trade Typesetting Ltd., Hong Kong.
Printed and bound by R.R. Donnelley & Sons Company, Harrisonburg, Virginia.
Printed in the United States of America.

9 8 7 6 5 4 3 2 1

ISBN 0-387-96642-0 Springer-Verlag New York Berlin Heidelberg
ISBN 0-540-96642-0 Springer-Verlag Berlin Heidelberg New York

Acknowledgments

The author wishes to acknowledge the assistance provided by the Dental
Health Education and Research Foundation of the University of Sydney, in
particular the active encouragement of the Foundation's Executive Director,
James E. Woolley. Thanks are also due to Ena Nomme, who acted as the
research assistant for this project; Les Wozniczka, who provided statistical
and computing assistance; and to Louise Kahabka, who expertly produced
the various drafts of the manuscript.

The manuscript was completed during the author's tenure as a Visiting
Scholar at the University of Cambridge. I would like to thank Colin Fraser of
the Social and Political Sciences Committee for providing office space, helpful professional advice, and friendly personal support; and to the Master and
Fellows of St. Edmund's College, where I lived for six months in a warmly
accepting and intellectually stimulating collegiate environment.

Contents

Part I
The Interpersonal Dynamics of Dentistry

1

Introduction and Overview: Issues and Concepts

In this chapter, the major issues, concepts, and research traditions that have been employed in studying the dentist-patient relationship will be previewed. Later in the book, these topics will be explored in greater detail.

Attendance Patterns

In western culture, practically everyone receives dental treatment at some point in their lives. However, the frequency of visits to the dentist varies greatly, the rate depending on a number of variables that will be reviewed in Chapter 2. These include patients' knowledge about oral hygiene, the availability and cost of dental care, patients' attitudes towards and perceptions of their dentists, and individual differences in the amount of fear that the dental situation arouses.

An important condition that interacts with the attendance rate is the policy of the dentist concerning the purpose and frequency of patient visits. Dental practices can be classified into three broad categories: preventive, restorative, and emergency. These three terms refer to the stated policy of the dentist, the emphasis that the practitioner places on the respective forms of treatment, and the most frequent style of therapeutic intervention carried out. In reality most practices will be mixed to some extent. Nevertheless, most dentists when asked will tend to describe their orientation in terms of one of these three categories.

Preventive Dentistry

Preventive dentistry, as the name implies, has as its main aim the prevention of dental disease before decay and other problems arise. Patients are shown how to look after their teeth, they are given advice on diet, and consultation time is taken up with cleaning teeth, applying fluoride, and other preventive measures. The dentist explicitly adopts the role of dental health educator, and a personal relationship often develops between the patient and the dentist. It is customary for patients in preventive practices to visit their own dentist every six months on a regular basis for perhaps two or three sessions of which one will be devoted exclusively to teeth cleaning and other preventive measures. The shared aim of both the dentist and the patient is that in due course the patient will attend surgery at stated intervals without presenting any major symptoms, and maintain that condition indefinitely.

Restorative Dentistry

A great many people do not visit their dentist on a regular basis (e.g., every six or 12 months). They only go "when there is something wrong with them," that is, when they experience a toothache or some other form of dental distress. Then they go the dentist "to be cured" of that specific complaint. It should be noted that the overall attendance rate of restorative patients is not necessarily lower than the frequency of preventive patients. For example, a person may not visit a dentist for several years, ignoring or adapting to the deterioration that is occurring, but could ultimately require a great deal of treatment often involving major surgery and reconstruction. Likewise, the overall relative cost of the two types of treatment is difficult to estimate, although it is probable that the savings made by not visiting the dentist every six months will be more than offset by the cost of the more complicated and protracted restorative treatment. The main difference between preventive and restorative dentistry appears to be psychological, and concerns the type of relationship between dentists and their patients. Preventive, health-educator dentists, who see their patients on a regular, fairly frequent basis, are much more likely to establish a personal relationship with them than restorative dentists, who only see their patients intermittently and under conditions of stress. This seems to imply that dentists in mainly preventive practices should experience greater job satisfaction than their restorative colleagues. However, the author knows of no direct evidence bearing on this hypothesis.

Emergency Dentistry

Finally, there exist emergency dental services, often operated by clinics and hospitals, and usually available at weekends and after hours. These facilities cater to people who need urgent, emergency treatment, perhaps after breaking a tooth, being in an accident involving the mouth, or suffering from an abscess.

Patient Attitudes and Type of Practice

As has already been indicated, very few dental practices belong solely in one of the three major categories. In particular, preventive practices may often perform restorative or emergency work. However, the main stamp of a practice should be readily discernible from the extent to which the dentist insists on regular preventive appointments.

The three types of dental practices are systematically related to two aspects of the psychology of the dentist-patient relationship. The first is the notion of *"my* dentist," in the same way as people come to regard *their* doctor, solicitor, or priest. It can be hypothesized that there will be a descending order in the extent to which preventive, restorative, and emergency patients respectively, develop a personal regard for their dentists. The second variable is the degree of enthusiasm (or reluctance) with which different categories of patients attend surgery. Again, a descending order of enthusiasm can be hypothesized for preventive, restorative, and emergency patients. The first of these hypotheses has received some indirect empiric support in a study conducted by the author, to be reported later in this book (Chapter 6). The second hypothesis has not been tested, to the best of the author's knowledge. These issues are important because of evidence indicating that both the nature of the relationship and the motivation to attend surgery, influence other patient variables, such as anxiety, the experience of pain, and the patients' regard for the dentist.

Patient Reactions

Very few people enjoy going to the dentist. Practically every patient experiences some stress. However, most individuals resign themselves to their fate, and enter and leave the surgery more or less intact psychologically. A minority, variously described as between 10% and 20% of the population, find the dental situation extremely aversive, and for these individuals dental treatment is a terrifying experience. A detailed review of the literature regarding attendance patterns and the incidence of dental phobia, appears in Chapter 2.

The reaction of the patient to the dental situation has a major bearing on the morale of the dentist, and on how easily dentists can perform their duties. Dentists do not like to be considered, or consider themselves primarily as inflictors of pain. Patients who fidget, squirm, and gasp with pain are more difficult to treat than individuals who accept the therapeutic intervention placidly. For these reasons, a great deal of research has been carried out into what determines patient reactions, with a view to reducing some of the more disruptive responses to treatment. Much of this research has been conducted by social scientists, or by dentists trained in the social sciences. Consequently, the literature has borrowed some of the concepts, theories, and methods prevalent in the fields of attitude measurement and personality structure. However, in comparison to the critical ferment periodically taking place in the parent discipline of psychology, there has been much less questioning of the concepts, methods, findings, and theoretical frameworks employed in the study of dental patients. A major aim of this book is to provide such a critical analysis and examine some of the assumptions that have achieved widespread acceptance in dental psychology, despite their rather sketchy foundations and lack of empiric verification.

Anxiety

The undisputed fact that most patients dislike dental treatment has given rise to several concepts and terms that are widely used in the literature, albeit with a variety of meanings. Perhaps the most common notion is that of *dental anxiety*, the idea being that the dental situation (i.e., the waiting room, surgery, dentist, instruments, etc.) arouses anxiety in patients. Studies of this syndrome will be reviewed later in this book in some detail. The anxiety is conceptualized as varying in intensity, extreme anxiety sometimes being referred to as *dental phobia*.

The concept of anxiety is frequently confounded with fear. As we shall see, some writers do not distinguish between anxiety about and fear of the dental situation. Others do make a distinction between anxiety and fear, and others still distinguish between rational and irrational anxiety.

A further problem relates to the role of pain. It is often assumed that anxiety is aroused by the experience of pain, or by the anticipation of experiencing pain. However, pain experience is a highly complex phenomenon, affected by a great many physiologic and psychologic variables, including the degree of anxiety present (see Chapter 3 for a review of this literature). It is therefore only partially correct to assume that pain causes anxiety because under low levels of anxiety less pain may be experienced. Finally, it is extremely difficult to measure anxiety, fear, and pain objectively, adding greatly to the research problems encountered in this area. We will return to these issues in Chapter 3.

Theoretic Frameworks

Perhaps the greatest controversy relates to the explanations that have been offered to account for the adverse reactions of dental patients. Major differences exist in the theoretic frameworks that have been employed to generate hypotheses, explain the results obtained, and justify the conclusions reached.

Three major, distinct strands of thinking have guided the research. The two most influential theories have been the psychoanalytic and behaviorist models respectively. The theories are similar in that both focus primarily on processes within the patient, but they differ radically in how the patient is conceptualized. As we shall see in Chapter 4, psychoanalysts tend to think of the patient as reenacting a childhood scene with an authority figure, the reaction of the patient depending on the nature of the earlier relationship. The behaviorists, on the other hand, regard the patient as responding to positive and/or negative reinforcements (reward and punishment), and whether a patient responds anxiously or cooperatively depends on the schedule of reinforcement operating in the dental situation. The application of learning theory to the practice of dentistry will be described more fully in Chapter 5.

More recently, a third theoretic perspective has emerged, influenced by developments in social psychology. The dentist-patient interaction can be regarded as an encounter that is subject to the same general principles that govern all social episodes, implying that how the patient responds will depend on how the various participants (e.g., dentist, patient, nurse, receptionist) perceive and relate to one another. Research stemming from this perspective is directed at the processes that occur among the various persons in the system and at the social system itself, rather than merely at the internal states of the patient and the dentist. The social psychology of the dental surgery will be the subject matter of Chapter 6.

The divergence in theoretic views is not just an academic matter, as the various theories carry quite different practical implications for the reduction of anxiety and patient management in general. A psychoanalytic perspective suggests that the patient's transference on the dentist should be resolved; behaviorists have developed various methods, such as relaxation, implosion, flooding, and systematic desensitization, which they claim can reduce anxiety, including dental aversion; and social psychologists maintain that a good, personal relationship between dentist and patient will reduce patient distress and anxiety.

The practical consequences of the theories will be a recurring theme of this book. In particular, the last two chapters, 7 and 8, address themselves explicitly to the question of what action is required in the surgery, training curricula, and research sphere if this literature is taken seriously. A major orientation of this book is to integrate theory with practical considerations. Theories that do not have reasonably obvious consequences tend to be of little interest to practitioners and are often intrinsically suspect because they are difficult to confirm or disconfirm. However, facts and figures that are not related to each other in some systematic way have equally little utility—they merely describe but do not explain the phenomena they represent. In this book, all facts, that is, all research findings or observations, will be placed where possible into a theoretic context that logically connects them with other facts; and all theories will be examined for their practical consequences in the day-to-day management of a dental surgery. This is a good way to keep both facts and theories honest: facts that do not fit easily into a theoretic system, and theories that do not have readily observable implications in the real world, often tend to be trivial, or at best interesting but not relevant to the purpose in hand.

Finally, most psychologic theories have some wise things to say about how people think, feel, and behave. Therefore, this book does not adopt a rigid dogmatic position. Although it is written from the perspective of social psychology, those concepts and practices coming from psychoanalysis or behaviorism that can be empirically supported have been described and commended to the reader. Where this book is dogmatic is on its insistence that all suppositions, speculations, hypotheses, and statements must be based on reasonably hard data, on the results of properly conducted experiments, surveys, and objective observations. This sometimes requires an excursion into the methodology of the studies being reviewed, particulary those reporting controversial results. Where a study has been poorly carried out, this will be pointed out, so that the conclusions can be properly evaluated.

Chapter 2 describes in greater detail the main psychologic parameters of the dental surgery as these have been listed in the literature. This will be followed by a chapter on the psychology of pain tolerance as it affects the dental situation. Next, there will be chapters dealing, respectively, with psychoanalysis, learning theory, and social psychology, and the practical implications of these theoretic frameworks on patient management. The last two chapters will offer an integration of the various points of view, a summary of those findings that have adequate empiric support, and the implications that can be drawn for the practice of dentistry, the training of dentists, and future research.

2
The Psychologic Parameters of Dentistry

The first step in any scientific endeavor is to identify and describe as accurately as possible the fundamental characteristics of the topic under investigation. This chapter reviews the many surveys that have been conducted to map the basic psychologic parameters of dentistry. The aim of these studies is primarily to find out what is the case, without necessarily setting the data within any particular theoretic framework. The surveys tend to fall into three broad categories: a) surveys of patients' use of dental services, knowledge of dental health, and their attitudes to dental treatment and oral hygiene; b) surveys of patients' attitudes toward their dentists; and c) surveys of the extent and degree of fear experienced by patients. Representative studies for each category will now be reviewed. The review has been organized around the question of why dental services tend to be underutilized from the point of view of maintaining adequate oral health in the community.

Use of Dental Services

About 90% of the population in western countries visit a dentist at least some time in their lives. However, only relatively few people develop or maintain regular dental habits. Kegeles (1974) has reviewed research indicating that in the United States, only 46% of the population visit a dentist at least once a year, and only 30% visit dentists routinely. Furthermore, the evidence shows a strong relationship between socioeconomic status and frequency of visits. Those who make fewer visits include underprivileged, nonwhite, older, and rural dwelling individuals. The pattern in Britain is similar: Richards, Willcocks, Bulman, and Slack (1965) report that only about 30% of their sample had visited a dentist in the 12 months previous to the interview. In a sample of 531 employees in two large London office buildings, Liddell and May (1984) found that only 44% of the respondents said they had regular check-ups, and 40% thought they needed some form of treatment. According to Lindsay and Woolgrove (1982), 40% of British adults avoid routine dentistry unless they are in pain. In Australia, Martin (1965) wrote that ". . . no one can state precisely how many individuals or what percentage of the Australian population receives appropriate dental care, there seems to be adequate grounds for believing that such care is restricted to a very small percentage of the population, and that adequate dental care is certainly not enjoyed by all of those who can afford it" (p. 9). More recently, Fanning and Leppard (1973) have suggested that about 30% of the general population in Australia, and about 45% of the university student population receive regular dental treatment. Higher figures have been reported by Biro and Hewson (1976), who conducted a survey in Melbourne and found that 66% of their sample attended at least once a year. They also report that females attend more frequently than males, and that attendance declines with age. However, attendance patterns are beginning to change, at least with regard to children. For instance Barnard (1976) in a survey of 1,895 Sydney children with a mean age of 12.5 years, found that 75% had visited a dentist in the previous 12 months. The introduction of the School Dental Scheme in 1973 (see below) has meant that progressively a greater proportion of Australian children now routinely receive a dental examination (Carr, 1982).

Another way to gauge the use of dental services is to assess the dental needs of selected populations. One of the most comprehensive surveys of this kind used a 10% random sample of all U.S. Air Force personnel on active duty in 1976 (Christen, Park, Graves, Young, and Rahe, 1979). The participants numbered 5,805 and the examiners were instructed to record the current dental needs of each patient. The results showed that each individual would require, on the average, 8 hours and 48 minutes of chairside care. Each entering recruit would need, on the average, 10 hours and 23 minutes of dental treatment. The clear implication is that these people could not have had a history of regular attendance.

In a dental survey of 620 Soviet immigrants to the United States, Ferber and Bedrick (1979) found that there was a need for extensive dental treatment among this group, even though they were mostly urban in origin and included many skilled persons and professionals. This study, too, implies a lack of regular attendance in the past, and reiterates the point that there exist large individual differences between groups with respect to attendance. Thus a different picture emerges in Australia, where a School Dental Scheme was commenced in July 1973. In the period up to June 30, 1981, almost 2 million examinations of children aged 6 to 13 had taken place (Carr, 1982). In effect, this group of patients has been required to participate in what amounts to a compulsory program of dental examination. Using criteria established by the World Health Organization, there has been a marked improvement each year in the level of dental health in the children examined, attributable in part to the work of the school dental service, to the progressive introduction of fluoride to the water supply of Australian cities, and to the growing use of toothpaste containing fluoride. Even so, in 1980, 34% of Australian primary school children had at least one carious permanent tooth, whereas 52% were affected by caries of either the permanent or deciduous dentitions. However, the implication is clear that regular attendance together with exposure to fluoride has a marked effect on dental health, particulary in young children.

Other surveys of dental health using the WHO method are now beginning to appear in the literature. For instance, the Pacific islands have been studied (Speake, 1980) as have a group of Australian Aborigines living in remote Mornington Island (Yule, 1975). These studies all indicate that there is a universal need for dental services, the degree varying with such factors as naturally occurring fluoride in the diet of the Gilbert Islanders, or the low consumption of refined sugar in Tonga, both places where there is a relatively low incidence of dental caries.

An obvious side benefit of surveys into dental needs is to suggest hypotheses about the etiology of caries, and to reveal correlations with incidence, such as the availability of fluoride or the consumption of refined sugar.

The conflicting results of different attendance surveys are almost certainly due to sampling error, such as using populations differing in age, when the survey was conducted and where, differences in socioeconomic status, and gender distribution. For instance, in a recent American survey, Chen and Rubinson (1982) sent a questionnaire to a stratified sample of 1,000 families, receiving a 71% response. Their data show that about 70% of the subjects who replied to the questionnaire had visited their dentist for preventive work within the year before the survey was taken. The authors conclude that this indicates that the preventive dental behavior of white American families has improved. However, the results cannot be interpreted in that way because it is quite likely that the 30% of subjects who did not reply to the questionnaire may be the very persons who do not visit a dentist regularly. Further, better designed research is needed to establish beyond doubt whether attendance patterns in the United States are increasing.

Few of the studies show what dentists would regard as a satisfactory level of attendance. This has prompted intense speculation about the reasons why patients do not visit their dentists more frequently. However, in this regard it is important to ask the right question. The question is not why people fail to seek dental treatment, as the vast majority of the population will ultimately go to a dentist if they are in pain. The real question is why people do not seek preventive care—why people do not routinely visit their dentist on a regular yearly or half-yearly basis. Formulating the problem in this manner suggests that there may be forces operating that either predispose patients to seek preventive care, or conversely, to avoid it. The forces are psychologic, because they consist of beliefs, attitudes, and values. Below is a partial list of psychologic variables that probably affect acceptance of preventive care. The statements should be taken as hypotheses because the empirical evidence is rather sketchy, and in some instances equivocal.

1. Belief in *susceptibility* to dental problems. People who believe they are susceptible are more likely to adopt preventive care than people who believe they are immune.
2. Belief in the *seriousness* of dental disease. People who believe that dental disease is serious, whether for clinical or for esthetic reasons, are more likely to visit their dentist regularly, than people who regard dental problems as minimally or moderately serious.
3. Belief in the relative *importance* of dental problems. People who believe that dental problems are important compared to other things that might befall them, are more likely to become preventive patients.
4. Belief about the *effectiveness* of preventive care. People who believe that preventive care works, are more likely to adopt it than those skeptical about its benefits.
5. *Perceptions* of dentists. People who evaluate their dentist positively are more likely to become regular patients than people who are dissatisfied with their dentist, for whatever reason.
6. *Anxiety* and *fear* of pain. Highly anxious persons tend to refrain from visiting dentists. However, studies indicate that only between 10% and 20% of the population are unable to tolerate the pain and anxiety associated with dental treatment (Agras, Sylvester, and Oliveau, 1969; Fanning and Leppard, 1973; Kegeles, 1974). Consequently, dental fear by itself cannot account for low attendance rates.
7. Perceived *cost*. People who believe that dentistry costs too much, or is a luxury, are less likely to obtain regular care than persons who regard dental treatment as a necessity.
8. General *preventive* orientation. Persons who have a preventive orientation toward general health matters are also likely to have a preventive attitude to dental hygiene; conversely, an absence of a general preventive health orientation may be reflected in fewer dental visits.
9. *Social modeling*. Important and significant figures in a person's life tend to be imitated and/or exert their influence on the individual. For example, mothers who obtain preventive care for themselves are also likely to obtain preventive care for their children.

The Evidence

The literature contains many surveys that touch on the issues listed. The main results will now be presented in summary and related to these questions. The scattered and unconnected data become comprehensible when they are interpreted against the criterion of whether a particular pattern is psychologically consistent or inconsistent with regular attendance.

Knowledge About Dental Hygiene

Several surveys of dental knowledge have been conducted, some based on fairly large samples. The results consistently indicate that the lay public is generally quite ignorant about dental hygiene. For example, in a New Zealand study based on 100 households, Bishop, Flett, and Beck (1975) found that half the sample thought that pregnancy increased dental decay, 75% did not know what plaque was, there was little knowledge about gum disease; many subjects thought that people are born either with good or bad teeth, and that oral hygiene had little effect on dental health. Similarly, Linn (1974) interviewed 105 patients in San Francisco and found general ignorance about plaque, flossing, and disclosing tablets. Seventy-three percent of the subjects did not know what the term "periodontal disease" meant, a word often used in dental educational material. In a survey of 2,530 American teenagers, Linn (1976) found that only 25% knew that periodontal disease was a disease of the gingiva; only a third connected sweet foods with tooth decay; and only six respondents knew about plaque. Brushing was the major oral health practice, but it was rarely checked with disclosing tablets, flossing was rarely done, and curtailment of sweet foods or drinks as an oral health measure was also rare. In an early study, Fadden (1953) found that 54% of his sample of 706 children, had not been shown how to brush their teeth by their dentists.

Dennison, Lucye, and Suomi (1974) have described a procedure for teaching dental hygiene that appears to be effective. The program took 10 hours to conduct, and contained three elements: teaching skills, providing information, and motivating the patients to use these skills and information. A control group received only about two hours of less concentrated dental health instruction. All participants were examined on a subsequent occasion to gauge the success of the instructional programs. Significant reductions in plaque and gingivitis occurred in both groups, but there was much greater improvement in the experimental group. This study indicates that under appropriate conditions dental health can be taught. However, many dentists might find it impractical to devote 10 hours to the teaching of dental hygiene. According to Chambers (1977), for most dentists the preventive component in their practice means providing a brief chairside explanation of plaque and its removal, with perhaps a demonstration or two. The evidence is overwhelming that this may be insufficient to change the behavior of most patients. This is unfortunate because there is no doubt that preventive measures work. For instance, in a Scottish study based on 161 children participating in a four-year preventive program, Donaldson et al. (1986) found that the treatment greatly reduced the incidence of caries. The preventive package consisted of personal health education, oral fluoride supplements, regular application of acid phosphate fluoride gel, and pit and fissure sealing.

Patients' Assessment of Their Dental Condition

Most surveys indicate that patients tend to overestimate the health of their teeth and gums (Bishop, Flett, and Beck, 1975; Richards, Willcocks, Bulman, and Slack, 1965). Ignorance about dental hygiene, in combination with an inflated estimate of the oral condition, can act as a deterrent to seeking treatment.

Attitude Toward Health

One approach used to explain preventive health behavior has been through the Health Belief Model (for a review see Weisenberg, Kegeles, and Lund, 1980). The model is based on the principle that people will be predisposed or ready to take preventive action if they believe that: a) they are susceptible to the disease; b) that the disease would have serious consequences; c) that by taking action the disease could be prevented or made less serious if contracted; and d) taking action would not be worse than contracting the disease itself. The idea that the health beliefs of a person might affect and predict their health behavior has generated a good deal of research in various related fields, including the predisposition to seek out dental care. The evidence, as reviewed by Weisenberg et al. (1980) is mixed, with some studies supporting the model and others not. The following study is an example of a report that did find some evidence in support of the model.

Gochman (1972) measured perceived vulnerability to health problems and perceived benefits of health care in a survey of 774 school children in the United States. Vulnerability was assessed through asking the children whether they expected during the next year to get the flu, a rash, fever, have a tooth pulled, toothache, bleeding gums, and so forth. A seven-point scale, ranging from "no chance" to "certain" was used to score the responses. Perceived benefits were measured by asking the children to complete the sentence "I go to the dentist because. . . ," and through items touching on appearance and health (e.g., "I don't want my teeth to look crooked"; "I don't want to have toothaches"). The children were also asked about their intentions to take health action, through the question, "What chance is there of your going to the dentist during this next year?," again using a seven-point scale. The rather complex results showed that perceived vulnerability and health benefits were positively related to the intention to visit the dentist. The investigator did not, however, directly confirm the findings regarding intentions against actual attendance in a dental surgery at a later date. This is a shortcoming of the study because a great deal of research in general attitude psychology indicates that what people say they intend to do, does not necessarily correspond with their actual subsequent behavior (Liska,

1974; Wicker, 1969). Nevertheless, the study does have obvious implications for health education in indicating that perceived vulnerability in particular, increases motivation to obtain dental care.

A more recent study partially overcomes some of the problems of the Gochman (1972) report by using a prospective design and a behavioral dependent variable. Weisenberg, Kegeles, and Lund (1980) gave 11- to 13-year-old children a questionnaire measuring perceived susceptibility (e.g., "What chance is there of you getting a toothache during this year?"); perceived seriousness (e.g., "Compared to breaking an arm, how bad would it be to get a lot of cavities?"); and perceived effectiveness of preventive dental procedures. The children were then introduced to a topical fluoride program and invited to participate in it. Compliance in the program was related to health beliefs. The results showed that only beliefs about susceptibility affected program enrollment. However, the results were contrary to the Health Belief Model. Thus a larger proportion of children with low perceived susceptibility volunteered for the program than those with high susceptibility. Similarly, once they had enrolled, low susceptibility children were more likely to stay in the program than children with high perceived susceptibility.

In evaluating these results it should be noted that the findings are unusual, although not unique (e.g., Bailey et al., 1981). However, on balance there are probably more reports that support than refute the Health Belief Model. Most of the studies that are consistent with the model were done with adults (although Gochman, 1972, used children) and it is possible that the theory may be more applicable to older persons than children, as it depends on the ability to make a logical connection between an antecedent and a subsequent event. As with other topics discussed in this chapter, more research is needed before the model can be discarded. In the meantime, its intuitive face validity suggests that it cannot be ignored as a principle when designing dental education programs, particularly as there is a good deal of evidence in social psychology that under appropriate conditions beliefs have a decided influence on action (Fishbein, 1967).

Rutzen (1973) found no differences between a group of 252 orthodontically treated persons, and a comparable group of 67 untreated individuals with malocclusions, on measures of self-esteem, courtship success, and anxiety. The only difference was on a test of self-perception, the treated group regarding their appearance as more attractive than the untreated group. However, this difference was not reflected in how the two groups of subjects felt about themselves. A possible interpretation is that people do not care as much about malocclusions as dentists imagine they do. The implication is that orthodontic treatment needs to be supplemented with explicit advice about the positive consequences of having better teeth.

With more severe deformities, the evidence suggests that restorative oral surgery can have a beneficial influence on the general well-being and mental health of patients. Marano (1977) has described the case of a young man who suffered from maxillofacial deformity due to an abscessed mandibular right molar. The patient was severely depressed and had been referred to the dentist by a psychiatrist following an attempt to commit suicide. After successful treatment, the patient's self-image and outlook on life improved and he became confident, self-assured and affable, saying in an interview that ". . . after 22 years, I now really know that I'm not funny-looking. It is kind of like having a new life and going into it with a new face." (Marano, 1977, p. 707). There is other evidence that individuals with jaw deformities are sensitive about their appearance, and such persons would certainly benefit from restorative surgery. However, the extent to which such patients are aware that they can be helped, is not clear from the literature. For instance, Marano's patient did not seek out treatment for his deformity but only underwent surgery because he was referred to the dentist by a psychiatrist.

Perceived Cost

In a Melbourne survey based on 541 respondents, Biro and Hewson (1976) asked if expense limited visits and treatment; 81% of the respondents said "No." However, when the answers were related to the actual frequency of visits, the data showed that those subjects reporting a lower frequency of visits were also more likely to answer "Yes," suggesting that cost does act as a deterrent. This conclusion is consistent with the outcome of other studies (reviewed in Biro and Hewson, 1976) in which lack of money is frequently given as a reason for not having visited the dentist during the preceding 12 months.

In an American study based on 838 respondents, Jenny, Frazier, Bagramian, and Proshek (1973) found that the primary reason for considering a change to another dentist was the feeling that their dentist charged too much. In another study done in the United States by Collett (1969), the chief complaint was that fees were too high. Things have not changed in the intervening years. According to Grembowski and Conrad (1986), for many Americans the cost of dental services is still a barrier to receiving regular dental care and maintaining proper oral health. Clearly, financial considerations affect attendance rates, particularly among the less affluent.

Traditionally, dental care has been financed through fee-for-service charges to patients. However, the past 15 years have seen the emergence of alternate arrangements, such as taking out dental insurance or participating in various prepaid plans. Strevel (1982) has estimated that whereas in 1962 only 1 million Americans were covered by some form of dental insurance, by 1980 the figure had risen to 80 million. One reason for this increase has been that employers often subsidize such plans for their employees, either voluntarily or as a result of industrial action. If the trend to insure continues and spreads, financial considerations may become less important as a factor in nonattendance, except in the case of obviously disadvantaged groups in society.

Socioeconomic Status (SES)

The bulk of the literature indicates that higher SES individuals tend to enjoy better oral health than lower SES persons (De la Rosa, 1978; Richards, Willcocks, Bulman, and Slack, 1965), and avail themselves more of dental services (Frazier, Jenny, and Bagramian, 1974; Kegeles, 1974; see also the review of the relevant literature in Biro and Hewson, 1976; Blaikie, 1979; Chambers, 1977; and Garcia and Juarez, 1978). For instance, Barnard (1976) found that lower SES children had a significantly longer average elapsed time since their last visit to a dentist than high SES children, and the low SES patients attended less frequently for orthodontic and preventive procedures and had more extractions than their high SES counterparts. However, Rutzen (1973) found no difference in SES between a group of 252 orthodontically treated persons, and a group of 67 untreated persons with malocclusions.

Jenny, Frazier, Bagramian, and Proshek (1973) found that lower SES patients showed greater fear of dental treatment, expressed more dissatisfaction with the personal characteristics of the dentist, and thought the dentist to be less competent, than higher SES patients. However, Wright, Alpern, and Leake (1973a) found no relationship between SES and cooperative behavior in child patients.

Although not directly a function of SES, King and Tucker (1973) found a significantly higher incidence of attrition among alcoholics than nonalcoholics, based on a sample of 347 male subjects in each condition.

Ethnic factors also affect attendance, utilization, and type of service received, probably because ethnicity and poverty are often interrelated, particularly among minority groups. For instance, in a comparison of Mexican-Americans (Chicanos) and Anglo-Americans (Anglos) in Arizona, Garcia and Juarez (1978) found that Chicanos visited the dentist less frequently than Anglos, had twice as many extractions as the Anglos, and significantly fewer orthodontic and preventive consultations. Lawson (1980) found that white American children were more than three times as likely to have had a routine examination than children from other racial groups. White adults had less extractions than adults in other racial groups. These latter data are remarkably similar to the trend found in Australia by Barnard (1976) that type of service tends to vary with the SES of the patient. Linn (1976) reported a similar trend in a survey of 2,530 white American teenagers.

The bulk of the evidence supports the conclusion that oral health and attendance are positively related to the socioeconomic status of the patient. Level of education (Lawson, 1980) seems to be the major contributing factor.

The relationship between oral health and SES can be put into the context of a positive association between general and not just dental health and social class. For instance, in Britain occupational class (whether of self, father, or husband) has repeatedly been shown to be associated with a diverse collection of health measures, including death from all causes, physical and mental illness, height, weight for height, birth weight, blood pressure, dental condition, ability to conceive, and self-perceived health (MacIntyre, 1986). Likewise, Lundberg (1986) found clear class gradients in health in both Britain and Sweden. However, the health gradient was steeper in Britain than in Sweden, reflecting the greater stratification of British society, indirectly providing further evidence for the existence of class inequalities in health.

Attitude Toward Dentists

In an early study, Fadden (1953) questioned 706 elementary school children about their likes and dislikes in the dental domain. The major preferences included the availability of a signal to stop the dentist, and the dentist explaining the function of the instruments and how they were going to be used. The number of children who preferred to be alone with the dentist, was about the same as the proportion who wanted to have their mother or father in the operating room, and the number who liked to go to the dentist was about the same as the number of children who disliked the visit.

In a Dutch study based on 513 randomly selected persons from one of the districts in Amsterdam, (Van Groenestijn et al., 1980a, b), respondents were asked to list the three most important characteristics of an "ideal" dentist. Professional skill, reassurance and the ability to put the patient at ease, and friendliness were the three attributes of the ideal dentist mentioned most frequently. However, there were social class differences: lower SES respondents valued reassurance and friendliness more, whereas higher SES respondents regarded professional skill and explanation and information giving as more important. The subjects were also given a questionnaire containing 22 statements about dentists and dentistry. In general, the respondents did not perceive dentists as caring, helping people, instead regarding them as remote and primarily interested in money. Nevertheless, most subjects had confidence in their dentists' capacity to deal with their problems. The special contribution of this study is to reveal that a discrepancy exists between how people expect dentists to behave (the ideal dentist) and how they actually perceive the behavior of dentists. This discrepancy relates to the social rather than the technical skills of dentists and could be reduced by practitioners developing a more personal, caring style in relating to their patients.

Studies have also been conducted regarding the characteristics of the "ideal" patient from the dentists' point of view. O'Shea, Corah, and Ayer (1983) asked 628 general practitioners to list the characteristics of the "good dental patient." The most often mentioned were concern about oral health, respect for the dentist's opinion, and being on time for appointments. In other words, the dentists valued dental sophistication and compliance in their clients. Thus, the good patient is the manageable one. This study again points to the problem already discussed, namely that persuading patients to become more manageable requires interpersonal as well as surgical skills.

Simply deploring the lack of cooperativeness in patients will not make them "better" ones.

In an American study (Rankin and Harris, 1985), 258 dental patients were asked to rate eight aspects of dental treatment. Patients liked having the dentist explain the treatment fully, explain the use of the equipment, explain how to act, and be truthful about the amount of discomfort to expect. Patients disliked having a dentist start treatment without explanations, tell them that a procedure that is actually painful will not hurt, scold them for poor oral hygiene, and fail to comment on their cooperativeness. Patients also reported that their present dentists' procedures were significantly more in tune with their preferences than were the behaviors of their previous dentist, thus establishing a link between the attitudes of the patients and their willingness to accept dental treatment. The finding that a majority of the patients preferred their dentists to be informative and truthful, is consistent with the results of other studies, and is incidentally one aspect of patient management that is relatively easy to introduce into the surgery because it is entirely under the control of the dentist.

Biro and Hewson (1976) in a Melbourne study based on 541 respondents found that in general patients had high confidence in their dentists. However, regular attendance and favorable attitudes toward the dentist were related. Of those who admired their dentist, 82% attended at least once a year, as did 78% of those with high confidence in their dentist, and 77% of those who thought their dentist was interested in them. By contrast, only 24% of those who had no confidence in their dentist, and only 30% of those who regarded their dentist as being rude, attended at least once a year.

In an American study based on 487 subjects, Kleinknecht, Klepac, and Alexander (1973) found that patients who reacted adversely to dental work, often attributed such reactions to a personal dislike of their dentist. Subjects who had positive conceptions about dentistry, most frequently cited personal liking for their dentists as a contributing reason. The evidence clearly indicates that the personal attributes of the dentist affect patient attendance. In a recent review of the relevant literature, Estabrook, Zapka, and Lubin (1980) concluded that visits and compliance with clinical advice are closely related to the perceptions of the practitioner and the delivery system.

Practitioners differ on how they should dress in the surgery. Some believe that they will make their patients feel more at ease if they are informally attired. Others consider that they will make a better impression by presenting a professional appearance, and accordingly dress in a clinical uniform. Cohen (1973) conducted an experiment to test these hypotheses. He presented 300 children with sets of three photographs. One was of a man in a jacket, shirt, and tie; one of a man in a shirt and tie only; and one of a man in the conventional white clinic smock. Equal numbers of boys and girls participated in the study. Half of the children were asked: "How would you like your dentist to look? Choose one [picture]." The rest of the children were asked: "Whom do you want to take care of your teeth? Choose one." The results showed no significant differences in the preferences of the children for any of the dress styles. Cohen concluded that the dress of the dentist probably has more effect on the dentist than on the child patient.

Patient Satisfaction

Weinstein, Smith, and Bartlett (1971), in an American study based on 1,048 patients, found that in the main patients were satisfied with the treatment they received. Patient dissatisfaction was positively correlated with dental anxiety and discontinuation of treatment. In another American study, Jenny, Frazier, Bagramian, and Proshek (1973) surveyed the parents of 838 fourth-grade children. Ninety-one percent of the parents thought their current dentist was good, and 80% had not considered changing to another dentist. Professional competence was the most frequently cited reason (52%) for satisfaction, followed by the dentist's ability to relate to children (37%), and the personal characteristics of the dentist (34%). Only 2% of the parents listed preventive procedures employed by the dentist as a source of satisfaction. Dissatisfaction was related mainly to feelings that the dentist charged too much, and doubts about the dentist's professional competence. There was also a tendency for lower SES patients to be less satisfied generally than higher SES patients. This study suggests that the public is insufficiently informed, or skeptical about the benefits of preventive dentistry.

Attitudes of Dentists

Martin (1970) sent a questionnaire to 310 randomly selected dentists in New South Wales, Australia. The final data are based on 182 usable questionnaires, or 59% of the sample. The main results, in summary, are as follows. A majority of the dentists think that the public have a high opinion of their profession; 85% consider dentistry to be emotionally exhausting but nevertheless, most enjoy their work, particulary procedures that show immediate results. Only 8% listed preventive dentistry as the aspect of their work they most enjoyed. Included among the items some dentists dislike, was treating children, dealing with nervous adults, and patients neglecting their teeth. Mechanical skills and technical competence were valued over sensitivity to people and powers of persuasion. Asked about the adequacy of their training, 93% stated that they were inadequately trained in managing their practices; 58% and 52% respectively said that their training in handling children and adults was inadequate. The areas that they felt they were adequately trained in were prosthetic dentistry (89%), oral surgery (66%), and preventive dentistry (66%). Blandford and Dane (1981) asked 33 dentists to list the problems they faced. The respondents described 324 individual problems. About a third involved the human relations aspect of dental practice, 40% concerned the management of the administrative and operational side of the practice, and only a fourth of the problems were concerned with technical or clinical difficulties.

In an American study, Corah, O'Shea, and Ayer (1985) administered a questionnaire to 746 dentists regarding how they managed their anxious patients. Seventy-five percent of the dentists agreed that "patient anxiety is the greatest barrier to people getting adequate dental care," and 78% agreed that "alleviating a patient's anxiety is the most important factor in the patient's satisfaction with a dentist." When asked if they treated anxious patients any differently from those not perceived as anxious, 83% said yes. When asked how, a variety of methods were mentioned including sedation. However, by far the most frequently used technique was talking to the patients, and most of the dentists believed that talking to anxious patients was worthwhile. But when asked how they had learned what to say to anxious clients, 74% said by trial and error, and only 23% from a course in a dental school. Finally, 80% of the dentists admitted that they themselves became anxious when working with anxious patients. This study further confirms that placing a greater emphasis on formal behavioral management training in dental schools and/or continuing education courses would be desirable, and would be regarded as such by the dentists themselves.

In a survey of 105 American dentists, Weinstein, Milgrom, Ratener, Read, and Morrison (1978) found that most of the respondents saw their patients as cooperative but perceived some difficulty in getting patients to accept and pay for optimal treatment, and to perform adequate home care or follow recommendations about dental hygiene. These data indicate that dentists seem to be aware that they are not performing effectively as health educators, independent evidence of which was presented earlier in this chapter. The study also presents some evidence that dentists tend to provide a higher level of service to those patients whom they see as appreciating dental care than to patients perceived as not being appreciative.

In an interesting longitudinal study of dentists' attitudes toward their profession, Eli (1984) followed 40 dental students in Jerusalem from the time they were admitted to their course, through their period of study, to eight years after graduation. Subjects were given a questionnaire prior to admission, at the end of years 4, 5, and 6 of their course, and again eight years later. The results are rather complex, but of relevance to the discussion in this section is the finding that when asked what rewards they could expect from their chosen profession, "interest in work" and "high income" were rated above "opportunity to help others." In other words, personal satisfaction was seen as more achievable (and perhaps also valued more) than interpersonal rewards.

The general picture that emerges suggests that most dentists are quite confident about the technical aspects of dentistry but that many experience stress in regard to the interpersonal side of their profession. Specifically, they feel inadequate about managing their patients and their practice. This is not altogether surprising because their training emphasizes technical competence and tends to give little weight to teaching interpersonal skills (Deneen, Heid, and Smith, 1973) or business management. A survey of 1,880 American dentists by Collett (1969) found similar results. Most dentists were satisfied with their profession but about half of the respondents had lost patients due to poor interpersonal relations.

Surveys of dentists are useful in providing information regarding the relevance and possible shortcomings of training curricula. They also confirm the perceptions of many patients that their dentists are cold and impersonal (e.g., Collett, 1969; Kleinknecht, Klepac, and Alexander, 1973). Finally, the Martin (1970) report in particular suggests that the dentists themselves may be contributing to lower attendance rates by implicitly denigrating the practice of preventive dentistry.

Included in a survey of 176 Australian dentists by Gaffney, Foenander, Reade, and Burrows (1981), there was a question asking if they were anxious while undergoing dental treatment. Fifty-eight percent replied in the affirmative, indicating that dental practitioners consider treatment to be as anxiety provoking as does the general public. These data can be taken to imply that dentists probably experience some stress while carrying out their procedures; not only can dentists directly observe the tension in their clients, but many are obviously also empathizing with the anxiety of their patients.

In a British study, Freeman (1985) administered a variety of psychologic tests to 99 clinical dental students and found them to be more anxious than the general population.

In an American study by Johnson, Pinkham, and Kerber (1979), dentists with varying degrees of experience were shown 15 slides comprising a range of potentially stressing pedodontic situations. Stress was measured by means of a voice analysis reflecting the degree of suppression of the micromuscle tremor. The results showed that higher levels of dental experience and education do not reduce the amount of stress experienced when confronted with difficult periododontic situations. This finding is interesting in that it suggests that dentists do not necessarily habituate to the less pleasant aspects of their profession.

There is some independent evidence that dentistry is a relatively stressful occupation. Cutright, Carpenter, Tsaknis, and Lyon (1977) measured the blood pressures of 856 American dentists, finding higher average systolic and diastolic pressures than in the general population. On the other hand, a detailed and exhaustive study of the mortality of dentists in the United States (Bureau of Economic Research and Statistics, 1975) found that for all causes of death, mean age at death was *not* higher for dentists than for the white male population. Further research is needed to establish the *relative* stressfulness of dentistry as an occupation.

In a recent British study (Cooper, Watts, and Kelly, 1987), a random sample of 484 general dental practitioners responded to a questionnaire measuring job satisfaction, mental health and well-being, and work-related stressors. About a third of the sample expressed dissatisfaction with their job, which according to the authors is two or three times the rate that would normally be expected in an equivalent white collar professional group. The main stressors were time and scheduling problems, and difficult patients (see also the discussion on page 151). On the mental health measure, the dentists scored significantly lower (i.e., showed greater ill-health) than a normative population of randomly selected general medical practitioners. There were also sex differences, with the male dentists showing lower psychologic well-being than the females. These data are suggestive but until they can be placed into the context of a systematic comparative analysis of stressful occupations (e.g., teachers, air traffic controllers, police officers), it is difficult to draw any solid conclusions. Nevertheless, to the extent that certain aspects of practicing dentistry are stressful, some stress management training for the profession, either in the dental curriculum, and/or as part of a continuing education program, would certainly not go amiss.

Women in Dentistry

Three questions arise in connection with the status of women in dentistry: how patients regard women dentists, how male dentists regard female colleagues, and how female dentists regard themselves. There is some evidence on each of these issues.

White, Betz, and Beck (1982) surveyed 95 male and 93 female patients. Half of the subjects were asked to describe the personality characteristics of female dentists, and the other half described the personality characteristics of male dentists. This was done by presenting subjects with 20 masculine and 19 feminine characteristics (as established in previous research by Bem, 1974). Subjects were asked to rate the traits on the extent to which these characterized either male or female dentists.

The results showed that female dentists were perceived as possessing significantly higher levels of some of the traditional feminine qualities such as being more cheerful, affectionate, understanding, compassionate and tender, than male dentists. Female dentists were also perceived as more likely to be interrupted by family responsibilities. However, the important finding was that female dentists were not described as less competent than male dentists. There were no major differences due to the sex of the respondent. Both male and female subjects described female dentists as equally self-reliant, competent, and forceful in comparison to male practitioners. Thus, females were perceived as retaining their feminine qualities while at the same time possessing the competence that is required to be an effective dentist. It should be noted that the respondents to this survey were relatively well educated, and further research is needed to establish the generality of these findings.

Quinn (1977) sent a questionnaire to 300 male general practitioners in New Jersey, receiving 154 replies. The topic of the survey was whether the respondents would employ female dentists and under what conditions. The results showed that most respondents did not consider the gender of an applicant to be important for the employment of an associate; that they would pay a female at the same rate as a male; that both males and females would be similarly restricted in the services they would be allowed to offer, the deciding factor being experience; and that competence rather than the gender of the applicant was the main consideration. The results of this study, although encouraging, should be treated with caution for two reasons: the 49% of the dentists who did not return the questionnaire may have declined to respond because of an anti-feminine bias they did not wish to disclose; and it is a well-established fact in attitude measurement that subjects tend to give answers that are socially desirable but that may bear no relation to how these individuals will actually behave in specific instances (Bochner, 1980). In other words, even though these dentists said that they would employ women graduates as associates, there is no guarantee that they would do so when the occasion arose. The only way to answer that particular question is to do a survey of actual employment practices, to ask male dentists how many women graduates they are currently employing, not how many they would employ if they had a vacancy.

McCreary and Gershen (1978) asked 82 male and 23 female first-year dental students in Los Angeles to rate themselves on 10 personality traits. On only two of the traits were there any significant differences: males described themselves as more masculine and orderly than females. Women did not regard themselves as any different to their male counterparts on any of the 10 traits. This study is marred by the relatively small number of women subjects included in the study. Nevertheless, the results support the general trend in the literature that sex bias is not a major problem in dentistry, in that neither patients nor members of the profession appear to hold strong sex-role stereotypes about either male or female dentists. However, further research is needed to establish the generality of this conclusion, particularly with less well-educated patients and in cultures other than the United States, where affirmative action programs over the past decade have had an impact on both public opinion and behavior.

Dentistry and Consumer Affairs

Diagnostic x-rays are a source of potentially harmful radiation. Unnecessary exposure can be minimized by providing patients with lead shielding aprons during x-ray examination, and most pertinent professional organizations recommend that patients should be shielded. Despite this, many dental x-rays are administered without such shielding. This prompted a Public Interest Research Group in the United States (Greene and Neistat, 1983) to conduct a study that had the dual aim of assessing the extent to which lead aprons were being provided by local dentists, and to then encourage greater use of protective shielding by the profession.

All 16 dental surgeries in two small towns were surveyed. This was done unobtrusively—the dentists did not know that they were participating in a survey. Several times each week an observer would go to the parking lots of each surgery and record the license numbers of all the cars there. The owners of the vehicles were subsequently identified from the Office of Vehicle Registration Records, and contacted by phone. (The procedure used in this study raises obvious ethical considerations. However, these are outside the scope of the present review. A discussion of these issues can be found in Bochner, 1980). The subjects were told that the Institute was doing a survey of citizens regarding their experiences and satisfaction with dental services. A number of questions were asked, which enabled the interviewer to ascertain whether the person had gone to the dental surgery on the date the license number had been recorded. Subjects were also asked if they had been x-rayed, and if so, whether a lead apron had been provided. This procedure yielded 841 usable responses.

After 14 weeks, dental surgeries in which lead aprons were provided to less than 75% of the patients, received what the authors call "a specially designed feedback package" containing: 1) a cover letter explaining that a survey into the provision of lead shielding was under way; 2) a statement about the danger of low-level radiation exposure; 3) results listing the percentage of patients who received lead aprons at that particular surgery; and 4) a "respectful request" to provide maximum protection for patients, and a statement that the surveys would continue.

The results showed that the provision of lead aprons increased dramatically after the intervention, in one case from 8% to 100%, and several of the surgeries maintained 100% usage for the duration of the survey (60 weeks).

As consumer action groups grow in numbers and influence, dentists, other professionals, and providers of goods and services in general will have to get used to the idea of coming under such scrutiny. For a variety of reasons, both self-regulation by the professions and government controls may fail in providing adequate protection to consumers. This unsatisfactory state of affairs has led to an alliance between applied behavioral analysis and consumer advocacy that in the past had been confined to the commercial and bureaucratic domains, but is now beginning to spread into the provision of medical, dental, psychiatric, and other health care areas.

Previous Experience

In a study of 774 American school children, Gochman (1972) found that children whose last visit was traumatic, had a lower intention of making a dental visit in the foreseeable future, than children whose previous encounter was not traumatic. In another American study based on 487 subjects, Kleinknecht, Klepac, and Alexander (1973) found that 13% of their sample attributed present adverse reactions to previous painful dental work. Lautch (1971) compared 34 phobic with 34 control patients, finding that all of the phobic individuals, but only 10 of the controls reported suffering at least one traumatic dental experience during childhood. In a study based on 225 American undergraduates, Bernstein, Kleinknecht and Alexander (1979) found that high-fear subjects had more painful early dental experiences than low-fear respondents, although the absolute level of reported traumatic incidents was not very great. Thus, 22% of the high-fear respondents attributed current anxiety to a specific negative incident in their childhood, but only 6% of the low-fear subjects recalled such an event. However, Pillard and Fisher (1970) interviewed anxious patients who reported having had no more than the usual amount of pain inflicted on them in the past. And Shoben and Borland (1954) in a study of 15 fearful and 15 nonfearful dental patients, found no significant differences in the incidence of early traumatic dental experiences, although there was a nonsignificant trend in the direction of greater incidence in the phobic group. The evidence about the effect of past experience is equivocal and further research is needed before any firm conclusions can be drawn.

Fear of Dentists

Virtually everyone agrees that dental treatment is an anxiety-arousing situation (Ackerman and Endler, 1985). Dental fear has been the subject of many surveys. Several distinct issues have been investigated, among them the question of whether there are sex differences, what is the percentage of phobic patients, and what particular aspects of dentistry are fear arousing.

Gender Differences

Several studies have reported gender differences in dental apprehensiveness, the incidence being higher among females than males (Agras, Sylvester, and Oliveau, 1969; Biro and Hewson, 1976; Corah, Gale, and Illig, 1978; Fanning and Leppard, 1973; Kleinknecht, Klepac, and Alexander, 1973; Lamb and Plant, 1972; Martin, 1965; Wardle, 1982, 1984). Martin has attributed the higher incidence of female fear to an unconscious association between oral and vaginal penetration. However, a more likely explanation is that in western culture, males are expected to be stoic and in particular not admit their fears. Females, on the other hand, are allowed to acknowledge and express their feelings, including fear. The obtained sex differences in dental apprehensiveness may simply reflect culturally determined differences between males and females in the expression of emotion.

Incidence of Dental Phobia

Estimates of the incidence of dental phobia vary from 6% (Kleinknecht, Klepac, and Alexander, 1973), to 10% (Kegeles, 1974), to 20% of the general population (Agras, Sylvester, and Oliveau, 1969). In a survey of general practitioners in Washington State, Weinstein, Getz, Ratener, and Domotc (1982a) found that 6.5% of all children were perceived as problematical. Some of the differences in the estimates are probably due to the way in which dental phobia is defined. Most writers identify the same two attributes, a *feeling* of extreme terror and the *behavioral* response of avoiding dental treatment. However, there is a great deal of variability in the way in which both fear and avoidance are measured and indexed.

The measures range from the use of projective tests to the monitoring of biochemical and physiologic functions before and during treatment. Venham and his associates (Venham, 1979; Venham, Bengston, and Cipes, 1977) have developed a projective test of dental anxiety for use with children that consists of eight pairs of pictures. Each shows two boys, one happy or relaxed, the other unhappy, crying, frowning, or tense. The subject is asked to choose the little boy in each picture who feels most like he does, and the score represents the number of times the more anxious member of each pair is chosen. Presumably a similar series of items can be constructed for girls. Venham claims that the method has utility in assessing dental fear in children.

An instrument that is widely used is the Corah Dental Anxiety Scale (Corah, 1969), originally published in 1969, and in a more recent evaluation described as "... a reliable, valid, and useful measure of dental anxiety" (Corah, Gale, and Illig, 1978, p. 819). In a Dutch evaluation study (Makkes, Schuurs, van Velzen, Duivenvoorden, and Verhage, 1986), the scale was administered to 60 persons suffering from extreme dental anxiety, and also to a control group of 60 persons matched on age and sex, who were free from anxiety. There were significant and substantial differences in the expected direction between the mean scores of the two groups, thereby providing evidence for the validity of the Corah scale. It consists of four items: 1) If you had to go to the dentist tomorrow, how would you feel about it? 2) When you are waiting in the dentist's office for your turn in the chair, how do you feel? 3) When you are in the dentist's chair waiting while he gets his drill ready to begin working on your teeth, how do you feel? 4) You are in the dentist's chair to have your teeth cleaned. While you are waiting and the dentist is getting out the instruments that he will use to scrape your teeth around the gums, how do you feel? Subjects respond to each item on a five-point scale of relaxed to extremely anxious. Other questionnaires also have been developed. For instance, the Dental State Anxiety Scale has 20 statements all beginning with the phrase "While at the dentist I feel..." (calm, secure, tense, worried, etc.), and subjects indicate their state on a four-point scale from not-at-all to very-much-so (Scott and Hirschman, 1982). Another scale in use is the 20-item Dental Fear Survey (DFS) developed by Kleinknecht, Klepac, and Alexander (1973). The DFS was recently put under psychometric scrutiny by McGlynn, McNeil, Gallagher, and Vrana (1987) using 4,288 subjects. The results showed the DFS to be a reliable scale having good internal consistency.

Another approach has been to use biochemical or physiologic measures of dental fear. The problem is that traditional physiologic indices of stress such as the Palmar Sweat Index do not always correlate with verbal self-reports of dental anxiety (for a review see Keys, 1978). An unusual attempt to solve this problem has been to use body-fluid content, in particular plasma cortisol and saliva cortisol levels as indices of fear. Keys (1978) classified 44 children as either phobic or nonphobic. The parents filled out a modified Corah Anxiety Scale describing their child's attitude toward treatment on the four items of the questionnaire. After anesthesia, but before dental treatment was begun, 10 cc of blood and a saliva sample were collected from each patient. Only the anxiety scale successfully discriminated between the two groups of patients. Neither the blood-cortisol nor the saliva-cortisol scores predicted a phobic reaction to dental treatment. Thus the physiologic measures failed to identify the phobic children whereas the paper and pencil test did.

Of the various physiologic measures available, heart rate seems to be the most promising. Thus Beck and Weaver (1981) measured the blood pressure and heart rate of 24 healthy adult patients prior to both a low-stress and a high-stress dental appointment. A paper and pencil test of anxiety was also administered. Anticipated stressful treatment did not affect blood pressure, which remained stable. However, heart rate and self-reported anxiety did show significant increases before the high-stress dental appointment. Messer (1977) took a continuous pulse rate measure of patients undergoing dental treatment, over a period of four visits. Heart rate was higher at the start of each visit than at the end, and there was an overall decrease from the first to the fourth visit. The highest readings occurred just before local anesthetic administration, before injections, during handpiece preparation, and during early cavity cutting procedures. These studies seem to suggest that a large component of dental anxiety stems from the anticipation of presumably painful procedures.

An interesting attempt to overcome some of the measurement problems is Meldman's (1972) dental-phobia test, utilizing heart rate as the measure. Meldman tape recorded the sound of a low-speed drill (10,000 revolutions per second) and played the tape to both fearful and nonfearful patients, monitoring their heart rate during the presentation by means of a finger pleythysmograph. The procedure consisted of taking the resting pulse rate, after which the subjects listened to the tape of the drill. Thirty seconds after the commencement of the tape, the pulse rate was measured again. The results indicated that in fearful patients the heart rate increased by an average of 15 beats per minute, in comparison to an average increase of 4.3 beats per minute in nonfearful patients. However, the number of subjects in each condition was quite low—only 11 in the "afraid" and 14 in the "not afraid" group. Consequently, although this seems like a very promising method for quantifying dental fear, further research using a larger population is required.

Differential Fear Arousal

Several studies have attempted to determine which aspects of the dental situation elicit the most fear. These studies assume that patients discriminate between the various aspects and phases of dental treatment, and respond with different amounts of fear to them. The alternate view is that for most patients, dental visits constitute an undifferentiated aversive situation.

In an American study based on 203 subjects, Gale (1972) presented patients with a list of 25 items and asked the subjects to rate these on a seven-point scale ranging from "no fear" (1) to "terror" (7). The five statements highest in the rank order were: a) dentist is pulling your tooth, b) dentist is drilling your tooth, c) dentist tells you that you have bad teeth, d) dentist holds the syringe and needle in front of you, and e) dentist is giving you a shot. Gale also asked his subjects to indicate the general amount of fear they felt in the dental situation, again on a seven-point scale. He then divided his subjects into two groups, a high-fear and low-fear group, and examined the respective rank orderings of the 25 items. There was an extremely high correspondence between the two sets of rankings; high-fear and low-fear patients placed the items in practically the same order. These results indicate that the same dental situations evoke fear in high-fear and low-fear subjects alike, although the amounts of fear differ. This is a very important finding because of the implication that patients respond realistically and appropriately to those aspects of the dental surgery that are noxious. The data suggest that most people do not have an indiscriminate fear reaction to dentistry, that there is high agreement among patients regarding what aspects of dental treatment are particularly noxious, that as with most other human traits and propensities, there exist individual differences in the magnitude of the response, and consequently, dentists should regard patient fear as a normal, healthy reaction rather than as an aberration or expression of hostility.

In a study with a similar design, based on 487 subjects, Kleinknecht, Klepac, and Alexander (1973) found that the highest fear was elicited by statements about the sight of the syringe, feeling the needle, and seeing, hearing, and feeling the drill. Females rated themselves as more fearful than males, but the rank order of the most fearful items was the same for both sexes. The study further supports the essential rationality of dental patients.

More recent surveys reveal a similar pattern. For instance Scott and Hirschman (1982) administered four dental anxiety questionnaires to 609 undergraduates. The majority of subjects reported moderate overall levels of dental anxiety; nearly all subjects rated a few situations as highly noxious (e.g., the dentist is drilling your teeth); and nearly all subjects rated some situations as creating little anxiety (e.g., dentist tells you he is through). Wardle (1982) asked 50 patients attending a dental teaching hospital how anxious they would feel if undergoing eight different procedures. Extracting, drilling, and injections aroused high anxiety, whereas polishing, blowing air, and filling elicited low ratings. In a Dutch study based on 949 respondents, Schuurs, Duivenvoorden, van Velzen, and Verhage (1986) used the method of paired comparisons to rank the fear-evoking qualities of six dental procedures: extraction of a front tooth, extraction of a molar, cavity preparation without local anesthesia, and injection of a local anesthetic were most feared, in that order. The least feared procedure was restoration of a previously prepared cavity, the second least being cavity preparation under local anesthesia. There was good agreement among the subjects, and the two least feared procedures were clearly separated from the other four, indicating that these two items created relatively little anxiety in most subjects.

There is some independent evidence to suggest that routine dental treatment, although not perceived as absolutely painless, is regarded as relatively mild. In a study by Klepac, Dowling, Hauge, and McDonald (1980), 58 student volunteers were randomly assigned to receive an electric shock to either an arm or a tooth, the shock being presented in an ascending order of magnitude. Intensity of pain was measured by means of the Melzack-McGill Pain questionnaire (Melzack and Torgerson, 1971). A third group of 29 dental patients not exposed to any shock, also filled in the questionnaire after receiving dental treatment. The results showed that dental treatment was regarded as less painful than either electric shock to the arm or tooth. The authors draw the not unreasonable conclusion that routine dental treatment among regular patients is relatively painless.

This and other studies reviewed by Klepac et al. (1980), further support the notion that the stereotype of the fearful dental patient may have arisen in part due to the sampling bias evident in many studies of dental anxiety. Anxious patients who are selected for study by researchers interested in the phenomenon of dental phobia, will by definition respond to dental cues with fear and react with pain. Only when a random sample of the population is studied, or suitable comparisons are made with other potentially stressful situations, can dental fear be seen in its proper perspective. Thus, after reviewing 17 studies of the incidence of dental fear in children, based on more than a thousand ordinary patients, Winer (1982) concluded that relatively, very few children exhibit disruptive levels of fear, and furthermore, that anxiety declines with age from about 5-years-old onward. We shall have more to say about this issue later in this book.

Fuller, Menke, and Meyers (1979) wanted to know whether the size of the needle affects the degree of pain experienced. Six dentists (subjects) received a series of injections in the retromolar fossa, by 25-, 27-, and 30-gauge needles. The participants were not aware as to which particular needle was being used. No significant differences in the perception of pain were found among the three sizes of needles, suggesting that size does not seem to be a major factor in the pain reaction. It would be interesting to see whether similar results would be obtained from subjects who did not possess technical knowledge about dental procedures.

Another issue has been the length and timing of appointments. Lenchner (1966) has reviewed the pertinent literature, which is divided between those who assume that patients prefer longer appointments (say up to an hour) and fewer visits; and those practitioners who believe that many patients and most children cannot tolerate appointments that last for more than 15 minutes. Time of day for appointments has also been discussed in the literature, with most dentists preferring to see children in the morning. However, very few controlled studies are available to provide empiric evidence about the effect of various appointment patterns. Lenchner conducted an experiment in which he varied age (preschool, 3–6 years; elementary school, 6–11 years), gender of the child, and duration of the appointment (short – 30 minutes or less; long – 45 minutes or more). Forty children participated in the study. The behavior of the children was measured by a questionnaire administered to the parents of the child, and to the attending dentist. There were no significant differences between the children with long or short appointments. Age and time of day also had no effect. The author concluded that temporal variables play a lesser role in dental appointments than is generally assumed. However, the relatively small number of subjects in this study does not permit any firm conclusions to be drawn and further research is needed before the question can be settled.

Some studies have looked at the time sequence of dental anxiety. Lamb and Plant (1972) measured the level of anxiety of 40 regular dental patients during three phases of the dental visit: a) in the waiting room prior to treatment, b) while the patient was in the chair, and c) in the waiting room immediately after treatment. The results indicated that anxiety increased significantly from the "wait" to the "chair" phase, decreased significantly from the "chair" to the "after" phase, and that the level of anxiety after treatment was significantly lower than during the "wait" phase. Women experienced higher levels of anxiety than men in the "wait" and "chair" phases.

Pillard and Fisher (1970) compared anxiety levels of 272 dental patients sitting in a waiting room prior to treatment, with the scores of 236 college students tested when they were in a nonstress situation. The study found significantly greater anxiety among the patient group than among the student group, further confirming that the process of waiting to be seen by the dentist is anxiety arousing. Implications of this finding for the management of dental anxiety are that greater attention may need to be given to the waiting phase. The current practice of providing magazines and piped music may not be sufficient to counteract the aversive properties of the waiting room. Another neglected area is in the training of dental auxiliaries (Deneen, Heid, and Smith, 1973), whose demeanor can have a marked effect on levels of patient anxiety, not just in the surgery but in the waiting room as well.

The effect of sequential visits has also been studied, particularly with children. Some studies have found that cooperative behavior increased on a subsequent visit, others have shown no difference, and some studies have found an increase in anxiety and a decrease in cooperative behavior on a later visit (for a review see Venham, Bengston, and Cipes, 1977). The inconsistency in the literature is partly due to the usage of different measures of anxiety, and due to insufficient measuring points (i.e., most studies only compare the responses of the subjects on two occasions). To resolve some of these problems, Venham et al. (1977) studied the reactions of 29 preschool children on six dental visits, using four measures: heart rate, ratings of clinical anxiety, ratings of cooperative behavior, and a projective picture self-report measure of anxiety. The ratings were made by three judges independently viewing videotapes of the visits. No differences were found on the picture test. However, significant differences were found over the six visits for anxiety, cooperative behavior, and heart rate, such that the responses of the children became increasingly more negative over the first four visits and then became more positive over the fifth and sixth visits. Presumably, arousal increased up to a point where the child began to habituate to the stress, allowing the patient to respond to the dental situation in a more discriminating manner.

The Transmission of Attitudes

A basic finding of social psychology is that many attitudes are not acquired directly by exposure to the object, but indirectly, by conforming to a prevailing climate of opinion (Horowitz, 1965). As Allport (1958) has suggested, many attitudes are not taught, but caught. For example, most individuals have very definite views about trade unionists, politicians, clergymen, communists, and vegetarians. However, in most cases the people who hold these attitudes are not personally acquainted with large numbers of trade unionists, politicians, vegetarians, and so forth. How are such attitudes formed, then? Usually, by ascertaining what the general consensus is (Festinger, 1954), or by finding out how people regarded as important, significant, valued, or trusted feel about these issues (Katz, 1965).

The two-step model of opinion acquisition has received very little attention in the literature on dental attitudes. Most researchers have assumed that patients form their attitudes directly through interacting with their dentists, an assumption that needs to be tested empirically in the light of evidence about attitude acquisition in general. The exception has been in the field of child dentistry, where the obvious influence of the mother is difficult to ignore. For example, an early study by Fadden (1953) revealed that 23% of a sample of 706 children reported that their parents did not like going to a dentist. The hypothesis has suggested itself to several investigators that maternal attitudes and feelings may contribute to levels of anxiety in child patients.

Bailey, Talbot, and Taylor (1973) gave the Taylor Manifest Anxiety Scale (Castenada, McCandless, and Palmero, 1956; Taylor, 1953) to 80 child patients and also to their mothers. They found a highly significant positive association between the two sets of scores. Other studies have found a similar relationship (e.g., Johnson and Baldwin, 1968, 1969; Sarnat, Peri, Nitzan, and Perlberg, 1972; Wright, Alpern, and Leake, 1973a). However such findings are only suggestive because strictly speaking, they merely indicate that anxious mothers tend to have anxious children. The studies do not show, except inferentially, that mothers anxious about dental matters transfer these specific anxieties to their children, thus making them uncooperative patients.

To test the question more directly, Wright, Alpern, and Leake (1973b) conducted an experiment in which they attempted to manipulate maternal anxiety. One hundred twenty-four child patients and their mothers participated in the study. Half of the mothers received a pre-appointment letter aimed at reducing their anxiety. This was the experimental group. The control group did not receive any pre-appointment communication. While the child was being treated by the dentist, the mother completed the Manifest Anxiety Scale in the waiting room. The child's behavior was measured on a four-point rating scale indicating the degree of cooperative behavior exhibited. The results showed a significant association between maternal anxiety and uncooperative behavior, but only in the control group. In the experimental group, the group in which the mothers had received a soothing letter, there was no relationship between the mothers' scores on the MAS and their children's behavior in the surgery. The authors interpret these findings as evidence for a direct relationship between levels of maternal anxiety about dental treatment and their children's cooperative behavior in the surgery. However, when the authors compared the cooperative behavior of the children in the experimental group with that of the children in the control group, no differences were found. Nor have any data been provided regarding the relative levels of anxiety in the two sets of mothers. Consequently, although the design of the study is quite ingenious, the results are highly inferential and do not really support the conclusions drawn. More recent studies (Klorman, Michael, Hilpert, and Sveen, 1979; Klorman, Ratner, Arata, King, and Sveen, 1978) have found no association between mother's anxiety (whether state, trait, or dental) on the one hand, and measures of dental fear and cooperativeness in the child on the other.

Some investigators have approached this problem by trying to relate child-rearing practices to dental anxiety. In a study of 26 children aged 3 to 5 years, Venham, Murray, and Gaulin-Kremer (1979a) found a correlation between dental stress and aspects of the parent-child relationship. Stress tolerance was less when the home environment was unstructured (i.e., when the parents were permissive, infrequently used discipline, and avoided punishment or restriction); and where the mothers lacked self-confidence and felt inadequate. The children were also given personality tests (Venham, Murray, and Gaulin-Kremer, 1979b), which showed that greater dental anxiety was associated with lower self-esteem and higher general anxiety, traits that presumably reflect the kind of child rearing they were experiencing.

Studies that link dental anxiety in the child, maternal anxiety, personality variables, and child-rearing practices may ultimately resolve some of the inconsistencies in the literature. However, at this stage no firm conclusions can be drawn. Further research is needed to establish the relationship between maternal anxiety and the behavior of their children in dental treatment.

Parent's Presence and Anxiety Reduction

Some writers have suggested that a child patient's anxiety would be reduced if a parent, particularly the mother, were present in the operatory during treatment. This suggestion has precipitated a controversy in the literature (for a review see Venham, 1979; Venham, Bengston, and Cipes, 1978). Many dentists discourage a parent's presence in the treatment area on the grounds that it disrupts the dental procedure and provides an opportunity for parents to project their own anxieties onto their children. Others maintain that the mother's presence increases feelings of security in the child (e.g., Brown and Smith, 1979). In an American survey, Cipes and Miraglia (1985) sent a questionnaire to all of the 60 pedodontists practicing in the state of Connecticut, asking them whether they allowed the parents of 3- to 5-year-olds in the procedure room during clinical examination and treatment, respectively. Results showed that 71% of the respondents permitted parental presence during examination, but only 55% allowed the parents to be present during the same child's treatment visit. In response to the open ended question "Are there special circumstances where you prefer the parent not to be in the room?," more than half of the dentists mentioned when the parents interfered with management or prevented communication between the dentist and the patient. The bimodal response pattern in this study suggests that dentists are divided on the issue of parental presence, particulary when treatment as distinct from examination is being carried out; and that many dentists regard the presence of a parent as detrimental to patient management rather than inducing the child to behave more cooperatively. Clearly there is a need to establish the actual as distinct from the assumed effects of parental presence during treatment. Studies that have addressed this problem have produced equivocal or inconsistent results.

In one of the better designed experiments, Venham, Bengston, and Cipes (1978) videotaped 64 preschool children during a total of 207 dental visits. Three judges independently viewing the tapes rated each child on anxiety and cooperative behavior. The judges did not know whether a particular child was accompanied by his or her parent. Heart rate and basal skin response were recorded, and a projective self-report of anxiety using a picture test was also administered. The presence or absence of the parent in the operatory depended on whether either the child or the parent requested it. The 207 visits included 46 visits with the parent absent, 51 with the father present, and 110 visits with the mother present. Presence or absence of the parents did not produce any significant differences on any of the measures of anxiety.

In another study based on 89 children but where the patients were randomly assigned to a mother-present or mother-absent condition, Venham (1979) again failed to find a significant effect on anxiety due to the mothers' presence or absence.

What these studies suggest is that the presence of the parent magnifies whatever emotion is already pervading the situation. In other words, anxious mothers are likely to transmit this attitude to their child and thus increase the patient's anxiety, whereas calm mothers are likely to reduce their child's fear through the same process. Because both types of mothers are included in the studies, when the data are analysed these individual differences tend to cancel each other out, and hence no overall effect for mother's presence relative to mother's absence appears. This hypothesis awaits empiric investigation. If confirmed, the implication is that dentists should encourage calm parents to accompany their child into the operatory, but discourage anxious parents from the treatment area, a conclusion consistent with the social-psychologic model of attitude transmission.

Probably more has been written on dental fear than on any other topic in the psychology of dentistry. Our treatment of this important field has of necessity been selective. The reader wishing to delve deeper into this area will find excellent reviews of the literature in Ingersoll (1982), Lindsay (1984), and Winer (1982).

The Management of Handicapped Patients

Fearful persons are not the only major category of dental patients to pose a special management problem. According to Willard and Nowak (1981) there are an estimated 33 million people in the United States with disabilities of various kinds ranging from mental retardation and illness to a variety of physical handicaps. The dental needs of these people tend to be neglected, due to factors such as reluctance by some dentists to treat certain kinds of disabled patients, architectural barriers in the surgery, financial considerations, reduced patient mobility, and a belief that such patients may not be treatable. These problems are now being increasingly ventilated in the literature in order to improve the accessibility and quality of care for disabled patients, particularly children. For instance, Willard and Nowak (1981) have discussed the need for dentists to be able to communicate effectively with the parents of handicapped child patients. Watson, Brundo, and Grenfell (1979) described a program to train dental students in the treatment of disabled patients in general practice. Ettinger, Beck, and Glenn (1979) have listed some aspects of traditional office design that may have to be modified in order to accommodate elderly and handicapped patients, such as special parking facilities, wheelchair access to corridors, elevators, the operatory, and specially designed toilets and water fountains.

Beck, Kaul, and Weaver (1979) have estimated that about 15% of the adults in the United States suffer from depression, and discuss the dental ramifications of this condition, including the need for psychiatric or psychologic referral.

In a British study, Nunn and Murray (1987) examined 1,730 handicapped children, resident in 25 special schools in Newcastle and Northumberland. While the total caries experience of these handicapped children was found to be similar to that in normal children, more of the dental caries in the handicapped was treated by extraction or left untreated. The prevalence of untreated dental decay was much greater, and the number of extracted teeth was nearly three times that found in normal children. Thus the treatment needs among many of these handicapped patients were not being met. Similar results were obtained in another British study, this time in Birmingham, where Shaw, Maclaurin, and Foster (1986) examined 3,218 handicapped and 1,344 randomly selected normal children. The caries prevalence was similar in the two groups, but the handicapped children tended to have more missing and decayed teeth than the normal children. As in the previous study, teeth were less likely to be filled in the handicapped group, leading the authors to conclude that handicapped children are receiving less dental care than their normal counterparts, and that when treatment is provided it is more likely to be in the form of extraction rather than restorative care. The solution, according to Shaw et al. (1986), is not merely to increase the provision of professional services to the handicapped, but to give them systematic instruction in oral hygiene and self-care, in particular teaching them how to carry out effective toothbrushing and other preventive procedures.

Many handicapped children do not receive regular treatment because it is (erroneously) thought that their behavior or coordination problems makes the use of general anesthesia essential. The evidence does not support this reservation. Gurling, Fanning, and Leppard (1980) observed the behavior of 132 handicapped children during a dental examination. The results showed that blind, deaf, and autistic children were found to be more difficult to manage than children with spina bifida. Nevertheless, the authors conclude that the majority of handicapped children who can learn skills under the guidance of special teachers, are able to cope with normal dental treatment and can be trained to carry out oral hygiene procedures. However, the authors note that minor modifications of facilities may be required in some dental surgeries if poorly coordinated children are to be treated successfully. Indresano and

Rooney (1981) have described a successful outpatient program for residents of an institution for the mentally handicapped. Klinge (1979) has reported on a program in which 10 adult male schizophrenics were successfully taught the basics of oral hygiene. Thus when special consideration is offered, good results can be achieved.

The literature survey indicates that the successful management of handicapped patients requires special skills in human relations. In that sense, the needs of the handicapped patient are not different in kind but merely in degree from the needs of the general patient. Most patients are affected by the management style of the dentist, but this may often be obscured in routine consultations. However, the truth of this proposition becomes patently obvious when the patients are "special" in the sense of being phobic or handicapped. We can learn a lot by observing how these special patients respond to the interpersonal dynamics of the dental situation, on the reasonable assumption that what is magnified in these special circumstances will be reflected to a lesser degree in most ordinary dentist-patient interactions.

Finally, underlying the problem of communicating with mentally handicapped patient is an issue that is of general interest in social psychology, namely the use of different speech registers with different categories of listeners. There is quite a large literature in this area, which was recently reviewed by DePaulo and Coleman (1986). One finding of relevance to the present discussion is that people tend to use what has been called baby talk (BT) when addressing not just children, but also mentally retarded adults and foreigners who do not speak the language well. BT differs from speech addressed to unimpaired adult native speakers in being more clearly articulated, simpler, more repetitive, slower, louder, and more attention-getting. It is unclear what the precise function of BT is, for it could be either a way of achieving better communication with a listener who might otherwise have difficulty comprehending unaltered native adult speech; or the main function of BT could be to convey warmth, protectiveness, and social support, in addition to its utilitarian function; or it may be a way of distancing the speaker from listeners regarded as inferior in some way, as a means of putting people down and establishing one's superiority. Whatever its function, the process is virtually universal, in that most people use BT when addressing babies and non-babies who in some way resemble infants, in the latter case seldom realizing that they are using a special speech register.

Little is known about how non-babies feel when they are addressed in BT. The social consequences of register use is an important and growing field of interest in general psychology and is a topic that could easily be studied in the dental surgery, both with respect to doing basic research into the structure of different speech registers and their function, as well as using this knowledge to improve the management of patients with communication problems, particularly those with speech impediments, the mentally retarded, those too young to have learned adult speech, and foreigners who are not fluent in the language of their dentist.

Conclusion

Literature reviews of survey studies sometimes resemble the telephone book—they can provide a wealth of unrelated, often conflicting information that is difficult to interpret and even harder to remember. To overcome this problem, the present review organized the material around the question of whether the data can explain the reluctance of many patients to seek regular dental treatment. Regarded from this perspective, the surveys tend to present quite a coherent picture. The evidence indicates that most people possess very little knowledge about oral hygiene, suggesting that they would be unable to interpret the seriousness of their condition from their bodily sensations. This conclusion is supported by evidence indicating that patients tend to overestimate the health of their teeth and gums; and by data showing that individuals who regard themselves as being vulnerable to dental disease, and perceive dental care to be beneficial to health, have a greater intention to seek treatment than people who say they are not vulnerable and do not believe in the usefulness of dental procedures.

Several studies found that persons who believe that dentists' fees are excessive, are deterred from making frequent visits. So are persons of lower socioeconomic status, presumably because they are less able to afford the service.

Lower SES groups experience more dental disease and receive less dental care than upper SES persons, are apt to receive remedial rather than preventive treatment, are less inclined to adopt preventive habits, usually do not have a continuing personal relationship with a dentist, and may not get the best care from the dentist they visit.

Attitudes toward the dentist also affect attendance rates. Patients who admire, trust, and like their dentists, and are satisfied with the service they receive, are more likely to be regular in their attendance than patients with a negative attitude toward their dentists.

The most frequent reasons given by patients for being satisfied are the professional competence of the dentist, the dentist's ability to relate to children, and the dentist's personal characteristics. Dissatisfaction is caused by doubts about the dentist's professional competence, and by feelings that the dentist charges too much. Dissatisfaction was found to be related to dental anxiety and discontinuation of treatment.

Surveys of dentists indicate that they are confident about and satisfied with their technical ability, but find the interpersonal aspects of dentistry stressful. This reflects the emphasis of their training on technical expertise at the expense of teaching interpersonal and management skills. There is a suggestion that many dentists do not particularly enjoy preventive practice.

The evidence on the effect of previous experience on attendance is equivocal. Some studies have found that earlier trauma do increase anxiety and reduce the intention to visit the dentist. Other studies have not been able to find a relationship between anxiety and previous painful treatment.

Many studies have investigated the incidence and distribution of fear. There is general agreement that female dental patients experience, or permit themselves to acknowledge and express, more fear than males. Estimates of dental phobia in the general population range from 6% to 20%. Studies looking at the differential fear arousing properties of specific aspects of the dental situation have found that extraction, the drill, and the needle arouse the most anxiety, both in high-fear and low-fear patients. Studies have also shown that dental anxiety follows an identifiable time sequence. The waiting room produces moderate fear. The fear then increases during treatment, and in the post-treatment phase, decreases below the pretreatment level. Finally, there is a suggestion that maternal anxiety may be transmitted to child patients, in that anxious mothers tend to have anxious children, but the evidence about a direct relationship between the two variables is tenuous.

Taken together, the literature confirms that levels of patient attendance, fear, and anxiety are primarily due to the psychologic forces bearing on the patient. The effectiveness of health education programs depends on using strategies that are correctly grounded in the principles revealed by empiric research and we shall come back to this topic later in the look.

3
The Psychology of Pain Tolerance

The popular view of pain is that it is a sensation, caused either by an external stimulus such as heat, pressure, or tissue damage; or that it is due to an internal malfunctioning of some of the body's systems. Early research on pain reflected this conceptualization and a great deal of work has been done on nerve pathways, the differential pain sensitivity of various body zones, and the differential pain-inducing properties of various stimuli (for a review, see Weisenberg, 1980).

However, clinical experience in the medical, paramedical, and dental fields suggests that a simple model of pain as sensation is inadequate. Procedures that *should* hurt sometimes do not, and quite benign and presumably non-painful interventions may produce an intense reaction in some patients (Skevington, 1986). Why is this so? One explanation, favored by those taking a biologic perspective, assumed that there exist individual or racial differences in pain sensitivity. This view implies that there are some categories of persons who are constitutionally more or less sensitive to the effects of tissue damage. The theory certainly has an ancient tradition, harking back to the Stoics, a philosophical movement founded in Athens by Zeno in 300 BC devoted to inculcating an indifference to pleasure and pain. The modern word "stoicism" is derived from this sect, and it may well be that some people are constitutionally less responsive to tissue damage than others. But even if this were the case, it would not be the whole story because it is difficult to actually pinpoint those constitutional variables that either enhance or depress pain sensitivity.

Although most of the work on pain has been done from a neurologic or physiologic perspective, from the point of view of the health practitioner, pain is a psychologic phenomenon, to be understood and controlled at the psychologic level as well as at the neurologic one. At this stage, it may be useful to develop a working model of pain sensitivity that brings together the neurologic, psychologic and social aspects of the pain syndrome.

Pain as Sensation

Most pain has a physical basis, usually tissue damage of some kind. One has to say "most" because it is not always possible to specify the stimulus in clinical pain, and there are many examples (e.g., the phantom limb phenomenon) where pain persists and in some cases commences after healing has taken place (for a review see Sternbach, 1968). There are also many cases of psychogenic pain where the suffering has a psychologic and not physical origin (e.g., tension headache and myofascial pain dysfunction). It is essential to note that malingering excluded, we are not talking about imaginary pain. All pain, whatever its origin is real to the sufferer. For practical purposes, however, tissue damage is a major determinant of pain reaction. But, the *degree* of the pain response is not necessarily a direct function of the magnitude of the tissue damage occurring. A classic study by Beecher (1956) illustrates this point. Of 150 seriously wounded soldiers, only 32% wanted a narcotic for pain relief, compared to 83% of the 150 civilians suffering a similar surgical injury. Beecher attributed the difference in pain response to the meaning of the wound rather than the extent of tissue damage. In combat, a wound signifies a ticket home, whereas in civilian life, it means tragedy and appears to be associated with more pain. This leads us to the second component of pain, the perception, interpretation, and labeling of the sensation.

Pain as Perception

Most if not all pain-inducing situations have connotations beyond the tissue damage they cause. Beecher's study of pain in combat being regarded as a "blessing in disguise" is merely an extreme example of a process that underlies many everyday situations. A poke in the ribs from a liked person is perceived differently from a shove by a stranger or enemy. Self-inflicted pain such as hitting one's thumb with a hammer is not the same as being injured by another. Malevolently caused versus accidental injuries have quite different meanings. From the point of view of dentistry, pain undergone in order to treat or prevent a pathologic condition is different from randomly or unnecessarily induced pain. The list could go on, but the principle can be stated quite succinctly: whether an experience is perceived as painful in the first place, and the degree to which it is perceived as being painful (catastrophic trauma excepted), depends on the *context* and the *meaning* ascribed to the event. Most routine surgery induced dental pain is noncatastrophic and is therefore affected by this principle. From the point of view of the social psychology of dentistry, whether a particular procedure is perceived as being painful, and the degree to which it is so perceived, will depend to some extent on the nature and quality of the relationship between the dentist and the patient; in particular, whether the patient has confidence in the dentist, regards the dentist as competent, considers the procedure to be necessary, and likes and wishes to be liked by the dentist.

Pain as Response

Of special interest to dentists and other clinicians is the response that persons make to potentially painful procedures. In general, clinical pain begins with the tissue damage that is at times an inevitable concommitant of a therapeutic intervention. However, as most practicing dentists can relate, even this is not completely accurate: some patients will respond with an apparent pain reaction at the mere sight of a drill or needle, indicating that the pain response has become conditioned to the surgical instruments that produce tissue damage. It might therefore be more accurate to say that the general pain syndrome commences with the anticipation of tissue damage. At the other end of the spectrum there are patients who submit passively to quite extreme interventions without so much as a whimper. Most patients respond somewhere in between.

Several variables complexly interact to produce the response to a potentially painful intervention. The first is the perception and interpretation of the sensation. Studies by Schachter and his colleagues (Nisbett and Schachter, 1966; Schachter and Singer, 1962; Schachter and Wheeler, 1962), have shown that internal bodily sensations are labeled in part according to the social context in which they occur. The more ambiguous the sensation, the greater the contribution of nonphysiologic variables in defining it. A vague feeling of malaise can be labeled either as indigestion or stomach cancer, with quite different results as to how the sensation is experienced, the feelings it evokes, and the action it engenders. In the practical context of the dental surgery, a patient can interpret a sensation as uncomfortable, painful, or agonizing. Different patients may interpret a theoretically identical sensation variously along that continuum of discomfort-agony, and the situation is further complicated in that the same tissue damage may produce in different patients responses varying widely on the sensation continuum. These differences in patient reaction cannot be attributed simply to constitutional differences in pain tolerance, but are a function of the social psychology of the dentist-patient relationship.

The second major variable determining the magnitude and quality of the pain reaction is the definition of what constitutes an appropriate response to pain. Let us take the hypothetical case of two dental patients who have both interpreted the sensation they are experiencing as being of the magnitude 4 on a pain scale ranging from 1 (mildly uncomfortable) to 7 (agony). Individual A is a stoic believing that it is a sign of weakness to display emotion. Besides, the patient is fond of the dentist, does not wish to cause embarrassment, and therefore makes a conscious effort to grin and bear it. Patient A experiences considerable pain, but hides it and does not let the pain interfere with the therapeutic procedures in progress.

In contrast, Individual B believes that when a person is in pain, this fact should be communicated to the world at large, loudly and clearly. Besides, Patient B does not like the dentist, having a sneaking suspicion that the dentist is deliberately causing excessive pain. As an anti-stoic, Patient B gives full vent to an expression of emotion, at the same time gaining some satisfaction from having embarrassed and annoyed the dentist.

The response to pain therefore depends on how painful a sensation has been labeled in the first place, and on the definition of what constitutes an appropriate response to that level of pain. As with all behavior reactions, the final outcome is a complex interaction of internal (within-skin) and external (between-skin) variables. The major internal variables include physiologic sensitivity to pain and enduring personality traits such as stoicism, or its opposite, Szasz's (1968) *l'homme doulourex*, who makes a career out of pain. The major external variables include cultural definitions of emotional expression (Bates, 1987), the context of the pain-inducing situation, and the relationship between the "victim" and the source of the pain. With regard to the cultural variable, the evidence is unclear, some studies finding cultural differences (e.g., Zborowski, 1969), whereas in other investigations no ethnic differences in pain sensitivity were found. Nevertheless, there is some evidence (reviewed by Sternback, 1968) that in Jewish and Mediterranean cultures there is approval for the public expression of pain, in contrast to the Anglo-Saxon attitude of deliberately suppressing a display of suffering. There is also some evidence for the existence of cultural differences in pain as sensation. For instance, Moore, Miller, Weinstein, Dworkin, and Liou (1986) report that Chinese dental patients describe tooth drilling as a dull, short-lasting pain, in contrast to Westerners who describe such pain as being sharp.

Recent advances in theorizing about the neurophysiology of pain have tried to account for the empirically observed interaction between physical injury and cognitive and sociocultural processes, and their effect on the perception of and response to pain. The best known of these theories is Melzack and Wall's (1984) gate-control model, which proposes that a neural mechanism in the dorsal horns of the spinal cord ". . . acts like a gate which can increase or decrease the flow of nerve impulses from peripheral fibres to the central nervous system. Somatic input is therefore subjected to the modulating influence of the gate before it evokes pain perception and response" (p. 222). Melzack and Wall state that the degree to which the gate either increases or decreases sensory transmission is determined by the relative activity in large-diameter nerve fibres (A-beta, which tend to inhibit the transmission of pain signals), and small-diameter fibres (A-delta and C, which tend to facilitate the transmission of pain signals); and by descending influences from the brain. When the amount of information passing through the gate exceeds a critical level, it activates the neural areas responsible for pain experience and response. The hypothesized descending influences from the brain on the gate-control system can explain why cognitive processes such as ". . . attention, anxiety, anticipation, and past experience exert a powerful influence on pain processes" (p. 230).

Melzack and Wall cite an impressive amount of empiric evidence in favor of the gate-control theory, too technical to review here. Suffice it to say that the theory has both its proponents and opponents, and the last word on the neurophysiology of pain is far from having been written. Indeed, the title of their book, *The Challenge of Pain*, sums up the situation quite well.

Finally, to avoid giving the impression that tissue damage as an antecedent of pain has been completely forgotten in the rush for more complex and less obvious explanations, it should be noted that several studies have shown a correspondence between subjective reports of pain and objective clinical findings of a physical disorder. Thus Kleinknecht, Mahoney, Alexander, and Dworkin (1986) clinically examined 65 patients suffering from temporomandibular (TM) disorders. The patients were also asked to report the presence or absence of pain in 14 TM disorder symptoms. The results showed that as the number of reported symptoms increased, so did the number of symptoms found during the clinical examination, which incidentally was conducted by four dentists blind to the patients' symptom accounts. Thus levels of reported pain reflected the number of examination signs of pain.

The Measurement of Pain

There are many problems and complexities associated with measuring pain, and a detailed review is outside the scope of this chapter. Only those issues relevant to the earlier discussion, and as they relate to the dental situation, will be treated in this section.

The literature distinguishes between measuring the *threshold* of pain, and *tolerance* for pain. In the present context, threshold is the point on a continuum where a patient first perceives or defines the sensation as painful. Tolerance is the point at which the individual is not prepared to accept higher levels of stimulation, or continue to endure present levels. Again in the present context, both threshold and tolerance will vary between individuals for "objectively" identical levels of stimulation, depending on the conditions identified earlier in this chapter. There is also a distinction between pain tolerance and a *readiness to complain* about pain, as discussed earlier in connection with ethnic differences in pain expression.

The measurement of pain clearly reflects that pain is a subjective experience. In most measurement schemes subjects verbally rate their pain on some scale. For instance, Sternbach (1974) asked patients to rate their pain on a scale of 0 to 100, where 0 is no pain and 100 is pain so severe that the patient would commit suicide. Tursky (1974, 1976) used a four-point scale: 1) sensation threshold, 2) discomfort, 3) pain, and 4) tolerance level. Kent (1986) used what he calls a Visual Analogue Scale (VAS). It is 100-mm long, and anchored at the high end by "pain as bad as it could be" and at the low end by "no pain." Subjects are asked to indicate the degree of pain they experience by placing an "X" on the appropriate spot on the scale.

Clinically, pain is usually described in verbal terms. Pain has been referred to as burning, aching, stabbing, splitting, pounding, and nagging. The severity of pain has been described as intolerable, unbearable, awful, distressing, and excruciating. To make some sense out of this prolixity of terms, Melzack and Torgerson (1971) developed the McGill Pain Questionnaire. Subjects categorized 102 pain terms into three classifications: 1) words referring to *sensations* (e.g. burning, aching, pounding), 2) words referring to *emotions* (e.g. exhausting, awful, nauseating), and 3) words referring to *intensity* (e.g. agonizing, excrutiating, miserable). There was substantial agreement about which words fell into which particular category, suggesting that pain is a multidimensional concept with a least three principal classifications.

Clearly, "Does it hurt?" is not a simple or indeed sensible question because it can mean at least one or all of the following: 1) What is the nature of the sensation? 2) Is it in fact pain? 3) What kind of pain is it? 4) How intense is the pain? 5) How does it make you feel? 6) Can you bear it and for how long? In the dental situation, probably the nature and severity of the pain are the primary consideration of the dentist, whereas it is quite likely that the patient may be more concerned about the effect of the pain and its duration. However, this hypothesis needs empiric verification, as the writer has not been able to locate any research bearing specifically on this issue.

The Treatment of Pain

The distinction between pain as sensation, perception, and reaction carries over into explanations of pain relief, creating some interesting theoretic and practical problems. For instance there is controversy in the literature as to whether analgesic drugs work primarily in suppressing the sensation, or the reaction to it. Thus, according to Beecher (1972) morphine does not affect merely the sensation of pain but also the response to it—the patient may feel the pain but is unconcerned. Other writers prefer a more neurologic explanation of pain relief, and there is no doubt that in modern dentistry the analgesics that are used work largely at the level of suppressing the sensation. However, even in this instance that is not the whole story. The clear message of the literature on treatment is to underline the large psychologic component of the pain syndrome.

Placebos

Placebo therapy is a case in point. Beecher (1972) has shown that 35% of patients with pathologic pain obtain some relief with placebos, the greater the anxiety the more effective the placebo. The basis of placebo therapy appears to be the patient's belief in the practitioner's skill and care. This reduces anxiety and increases the expectation that the treatment will work. Clearly, the crucial ingredient is the nature and quality of the relationship between the therapist and the patient. It is likely that the placebo reaction is not just a rare occurrence restricted to neurotic patients, but is potentially present in all healing relationships.

In a review of the placebo literature as it relates to dentistry, Beck (1977) summarized the main factors that enhance the placebo influence. Placebos are most effective when the level of patient stress is high, when patients expect or anticipate relief, when the patient has had a previous history of successful medical or dental treatment, if there is a good relationship between the patient and the practitioner, and if the practitioner and/or the institutional context of the practitioner enjoy fame or high status.

There is direct evidence that placebos work in reducing pain in the dental situation, and that their effectiveness is a function of the dentist-patient relationship. For instance, Laskin and Greene (1972) and Greene and Laskin (1974) found that 26 out of 50 patients with myofascial pain dysfunction (MPD) showed long-term improvement after the administration of a placebo capsule dispensed by prescription and enhanced by a suggestive name. But placebos do not depend only on drugs. Goodman, Greene and Laskin (1976) reported that two mock tooth equilibrations for MPD produced remission of symptoms in 16 out of 25 patients.

In a review of the placebo effect in medical practice, Ross and Olson (1982) state that it is a very pervasive phenomenon. Physicians have employed placebos for centuries to treat sick people. Until relatively recently, most medicines had no specific pharmacologic properties that would alleviate the suffering for which they were being prescribed. A list of traditional prescriptions includes lizard's blood, crocodile dung, the teeth of pigs, powdered donkey's penis, leeches, poultices, and other remedies of little true value (unlike for instance citrus fruit, which was accidentally found to cure scurvy).

Although modern medicine has a firmer scientific base, substances of dubious pharmacologic value are still in widespread use. Vitamin supplements are a case in point. Ross and Olson's review suggests that up to one third of the drugs prescribed in the United States may be placebos, and in many societies folk medicine, medicine not supported by scientific evidence, is still widely practiced.

Research on the therapeutic effects of placebos shows that they "work" in alleviating a wide variety of complaints, ranging from radiation sickness, multiple sclerosis, postoperative pain, diabetes, ulcers, parkinsonism, to sea sickness, headaches, and the common cold. Naturally this has stimulated a great deal of interest in trying to understand the placebo effect and account for it, leading to a number of proposed explanations. We have already mentioned that placebos tend to reduce patients' anxiety. Perhaps worrying about a problem only makes it worse so that if a patient can be induced to become less anxious, the affliction may lessen. Another possibility is that after receiving placebo treatment, individuals will pick out and accentuate any small improvements in their condition that they would otherwise not have noticed, and that they will downplay the significance of any negative changes that otherwise would have bothered them. Similarly, placebo recipients may label ambiguous somatic sensations as an indication of an improvement in their condition, in accordance with their induced expectation of positive change. Another explanation states that placebo recipients simply comply with the demand characteristics (Orne, 1962) of the situation: patients know or infer the effects that the placebos are expected to have, and (mistakenly) for the sake of science, or as is more likely, in order to preserve a positive relationship with their therapist, will confirm the physician's expectations and "fake" their improvement. The forced-compliance paradigm (see discussion on page 139) would then account for any real changes in the patients' condition. Yet another speculation regards placebo reactions as conditioned responses, linked to previous experience with true medication. In other words, the pharmacologic effects of a drug can be evoked by stimuli associated with its administration through the operation of classic conditioning. For instance, hypodermic needles normally contain a drug that has some specific effect. It is possible that in some circumstances the needle by itself will become a sufficient stimulus for that response, irrespective of what is being injected. Genuine pills come out of medicine bottles. After enough repetitions, the bottle, through classic conditioning, may take on the properties of its contents, so that even fake pills will have an effect, provided they are perceived to originate from a "genuine" bottle. Finally, there may be individual differences in the predisposition of people to respond to placebos, some individuals being more suggestible than others.

This analysis of the psychology of placebo effects indicates that the recipients of placebos may anticipate certain somatic reactions because they believe that the placebo is similar to a previously administered drug and/or they are being provided with implicit or explicit suggestions about the impact of the placebo. These expectations will reduce anxiety and may under certain conditions induce actual somatic changes, incidentally an outcome in accord with the gate-control theory of pain discussed in the preceding section. Patients may also interpret ambiguous or minor somatic sensations in accordance with the expectations set up by the placebo procedure. Finally, to restate an important point made earlier, the effectiveness of the enterprise ultimately rests on the extent to which patients have faith in, believe, and trust their therapists, that is, on the quality of the therapist-patient relationship.

Hypnosis

Hypnosis is another successful nonphysiologic pain reducing technique (Finer, 1972). This is not the place to review the argument raging in psychology about the nature and indeed the very existence of hypnosis as a state (Hilgrad, 1973; Orne, 1976) except to say that it works (for a review see Sternbach, 1968). Countless studies have shown that hypnotic suggestion can relieve pain, among many of its other demonstrated effects. In dentistry, hypnosis has been used in the treatment of pulpectomy, pulpotomy, extraction, periodontal currettage, bruxism, tongue thrust, hemophilia, gagging, treatment of temporomandibular joint problems, phobias, and pain (Gerschman, Burrows, and Reade, 1978; Graham, 1974). According to these authors, hypnotic procedures need not be too time consuming or laborious in general practice. The authors state that a majority of patients are able to enter into a light hypnotic trance, which is sufficient to reduce fear and anxiety. In a study of 52 dental patients who received hypnotherapy, Gerschman et al. (1978) found hypnosis to be effective in reducing both psychogenic and organic pain to acceptable levels. It is unclear whether hypnosis works at the level of sensation, perception, or response. Hypnosis seems to be most effective with subjects who readily respond to suggestion. In social-psychologic terms, the effectiveness of hypnosis depends on the quality of the relationship between the therapist and the patient. As with the placebo reaction, suggestion is probably not a rare occurrence restricted to neurotic patients, but is likely to be present in all healing relationships.

Pure hypnosis may not be a practical solution in most dental surgeries. However, dentists by their manner and conversation can try to relax their patients, thereby reducing their anxiety and making them more receptive to suggestion.

Myofascial Pain Dysfunction (MPD)

There appears to be general agreement in the literature that the etiology of MPD contains a large psychogenic component. Likewise, it has not escaped some writers that if MPD is a psychophysiologic disease, rather than treating it purely with mechanical and biochemical methods, associated psychologic intervention may also be indicated. These ideas have stimulated a good deal of research that by and large shows that MPD symptoms will respond to psychotherapy (Pomp, 1974), group therapy (Marbach and Dworkin, 1975), a good dentist-patient relationship (Greene and Laskin, 1974), mock equilibration (Goodman, Greene, and Laskin, 1976), relaxation and EMG biofeedback (Gessel, 1975), and other psychologic techniques.

However, not all MPD sufferers respond to psychologic treatment. Schwartz, Greene, and Laskin (1979) compared 42 successfully treated female MPD patients with 42 unsuccessfully treated ones on a variety of personality characteristics. The results showed that MPD sufferers differ from the general population in scoring higher on measures of hysteria and hypochondriasis, indicating a greater tendency to repression and somatization. Within the MPD group the nonresponders showed a greater overall degree of emotional distress. Other studies trying to distinguish MPD sufferers from the general population have found that when exposed to stress, these patients respond with increased masticatory muscle activity rather than with a general increase in body muscle tonus (Mercuri, Olson, and Laskin, 1979).

Thus the MPD literature supports the conclusion that psychologic factors are implicated in its etiology and that psychologic techniques can enhance the management and treatment of MPD patients. Sometimes a general truth can be observed in circumstances where a particular feature is prominently displayed. MPD is such an instance. Without wishing to overstate the case, it is likely that most dental pain may have a similar profile, with psychologic aspects entering into its etiology and management. Consequently, the MPD model may be able to account for many other instances of dental pain, although only further research can establish the general utility of such a conceptual approach.

Preparation

Should patients be warned and prepared for a painful experience? The literature, and indeed the theoretic expectations about the effect of preparation are unclear. Some patients may prefer to be told about the nature and severity of the pain they can expect during treatment and worry less once they possess this information. Other patients may not wish to know, and the knowledge may increase rather than decrease their anxiety.

In some circumstances, patients may not remember or be receptive to the information provided. This was the case in a study by Herbertt and Innes (1979), who used 222 male and 200 female children aged from 5 to 11, to assess the effect of familiarization and preparatory information on dental anxiety. Subjects were randomly assigned to three pre-visit conditions: a familiarization group, in which the children were given a short lesson in dental health, and were then taken into the clinic operating room; a preparatory information group, in which the children were given a short lesson in dental health, followed by an inspection of the clinic *and* an explanation of the procedures to be used; and a control group that received only the lesson in dental health. No significant differences were found in the degree of subsequent cooperation exhibited by the three groups. The authors concluded that brief familiarization and lectures on what was to occur in the clinic is unlikely to have a substantial effect on patient anxiety, particularly in young children, possibly because these patients do not attend to or retain the information given to them.

Preexposure has also been tried as a means of reducing dental anxiety. The idea behind this method is that preexposing a child to a potentially noxious

situation may prevent the development of subsequent uncooperative behavior. In a sense this method is a variation of the preparation technique,
with the preparation consisting of behavioral rather than cognitive information about what is entailed in dental treatment. The method has been evaluated by Rouleau, Ladouceur, and Dufour (1981). Thirty-eight children aged
from 4 to 6 were randomly assigned to one of four conditions. In the one-film
preexposure condition, subjects saw a videotape of a dental situation. In the
two-film condition, they saw the film twice. In the in vivo preexposure group,
subjects were shown the situation directly in the dental office. Finally, there
was a control group, who were shown a non-dental film made for children.
Subsequently the children were given a dental examination, which was
videotaped. No significant differences on cooperative behavior were found
among any of the four groups. In a similar preexposure study by Fields and
Pinkham (1976), in which children also watched a videotape modeling cooperative behavior, no significant effect on subsequent cooperative behavior
was found. These results are consistent with other studies showing that
preparation does not seem to have an effect on dental anxiety, at least in the
case of mildly aversive procedures.

Another factor is the kind of information provided. A number of experiments (reviewed by Leventhal, Brown, Shacham, and Engquist, 1979) have
shown that some forms of preparatory information can reduce distress during
subsequent exposure to noxious stimulation, whereas other kinds of warnings
may actually increase distress. In general, three different types of information
can be given to patients about to undergo a potentially painful procedure:
a) information about the distinctive features or sensory properties of the
noxious stimulus, b) information on the individual's likely arousal and/or
emotional reaction to the stimulus, and c) information about the potential
magnitude in painfulness of the noxious stimulus. In a study that directly
compared the three types of information, Leventhal et al. (1979) found
that sensation information reduced distress more effectively than arousal or
pain information. Indeed, when a pain warning was included, the effect of
sensory information was negated and distress remained high. This study,
and others like it, suggest that sensation information leads to an objective,
nonthreatening categorization of the stimulus, whereas pain warnings may
arouse anticipatory anxiety about the forthcoming noxious event. Clearly,
the most useful information is that which helps patients to correctly identify
their sensations. For instance, debris in the mouth can be mistaken for tooth
chips, and the dentist should be able to reduce patient anxiety with information anticipating this sensation so that the patient can correctly interpret it as
a harmless consequence of the procedure. However, such information giving
will only be effective if the patient believes what the dentist says, which in
turn will depend on the quality of the relationship between them.

In a British experiment, Wardle (1983) assigned 73 patients to three conditions: *sensation information* (the dentist giving the patient a running commentary on the procedures and their likely associated sensations, including pain);
distraction (a visually interesting stimulus, Escher's Everlasting Waterfall,

projected on the ceiling); and *perceived control* (subjects were asked to raise an arm if they wanted a pause). A normal treatment group was also included as a control condition. After treatment, the dentists rated their patients' pain and anxiety levels, and the patients also rated their own levels of pain and anxiety.

Only the sensation-information condition had an effect on anxiety—patients in this condition being significantly less anxious than the normal treatment group. With regard to pain, both the sensation-information and the perceived control groups reported significantly less pain than the normal treatment group. Presumably the provision of continuous information about what the sensations mean is regarded by patients as credible and used by them to accurately label their sensations, thus reducing their anxiety and through this their levels of pain experienced. (The effect of labeling ambiguous sensations on anxiety and fear arousal is discussed more fully in Chapter 6.)

Postoperative healing

Recovery from surgery has also been shown to be affected by psychological variables. George and Scott (1982) have reviewed this literature, which on the whole supports the view that postoperative rate of healing and amount of pain experienced are influenced by patient expectations, levels of anxiety, preoperative encouragement and suggestion, group discussion, relaxation training, and reassurance. Again, these procedures are likely to be more effective if there exists a good relationship between the patient and the dentist.

Practical Implications for Reducing Dental Pain

In the modern dental surgery, the physiologic level of experienced pain, pain-as-sensation, is relatively low. Due to the use of sophisticated equipment and pain-killing drugs, the "objective" amount of pain inflicted on most patients should not rise above the discomfort threshold. Nevertheless, many patients experience high levels of subjective pain and/or give vent to emotional expression that interferes with the therapeutic procedures and causes distress to the dentist. What can be done to reduce these undesirable reactions? Let us briefly outline the implications for pain reduction, using the same categories as those that were employed in developing the model of pain sensitivity.

Reducing Pain as Sensation

Most dentists attack the problem predominantly at the level of pain-as-sensation, in effect trying to produce as little sensation as possible, through the use of sensation-depressing instruments and drugs. If pain were coextensive with sensation, going to the dentist would be rather like getting your hair cut. Clinical experience suggests otherwise, and provides evidence for the view that pain is not a simple physiologic reaction to tissue damage. Most dentists are already doing everything in their power to reduce pain-as-sensation.

Reducing Pain as Perception

The extent and degree to which a sensation is perceived or labeled as painful depends on one or all of the following:

1. The *confidence* of the patient in the dentist. Patients who expect to be hurt will interpret their sensations accordingly. Patients who lack confidence in the skill and concern of their dentist will expect to feel pain.
2. The level of patient *anxiety*. Research reviewed by Sternbach (1968) indicates that in general the greater the level of anxiety, the greater the pain experienced. Anxious patients are likely to interpret their sensations as more painful than relaxed patients.
3. *Past experience*. Patients who were badly hurt on a previous dental occasion are likely to expect to be hurt again (Lautch, 1971), and will interpret their sensations accordingly.
4. The *cues* available to the patient. Many of the objects to be found in a dental surgery look as if they should hurt, being sharp and/or cutting instruments. Often, the verbal commentary of the dentist reinforces this view. When a dentist says to a patient "This will not hurt" as a sharp instrument is introduced into the mouth, the patient may not believe the statement. To successfully employ suggestion and the placebo effect for pain reduction, dentists must use more subtle and sophisticated means than bald assertions that patients may have difficulty in accepting as true.

What can dentists do to reduce or eliminate the conditions leading to patients perceiving the procedures as painful? One clear implication is in the realm of the dentist-patient relationship. Patients who trust and like their dentist are less likely to expect to be hurt and hence less likely to label their sensations as painful. Such patients are also going to be less anxious and more likely to believe the dentist's assertion that the procedures do not cause pain. Also, to the extent that dentists can control the physical environment of their surgeries, they can choose equipment that is less suggestive of pain.

Reducing Pain as Response

The expression of pain depends on one or all of the following:

1. *Physiologic sensitivity* to pain.
2. *Individual differences* in the expression of emotion.
3. *Cultural differences* in the expression of emotion.
4. The *message* a patient sends to express or suppress a painful reaction.

As was stated earlier, dentists pay a great deal of attention to controlling physiologic sensitivity to pain, and short of applying a general anesthetic, cannot do more than is already being achieved. In any case, there have been warnings in the literature (e.g., Lambert, 1980) that the use of hypnosedatives may produce psychologic complications in some patients, such as drowsiness, amnesia, and anxiety reactions, so that sedation should be used only in special circumstances. Regarding the expression of emotion, in an ideal world all dental patients would be followers of Zeno and submit to their treatment with stoic determination. Indeed, the vast proportion of patients more or less do just that. The dentist probably cannot directly modify the behavior of the minority of patients who make an exaggerated and in a sense inappropriate response to routine treatment. Here it is a case of the dentist having to accept it because telling an adult patient that they are behaving inappropriately could be insulting, although it may work with children. In the final analysis, the relationship is again a crucial variable. Patients who respect and admire their dentist are more likely to attempt to suppress their emotional expression so as not to embarrass the dentist, than patients who are hostile. Positively inclined patients may also be more receptive to the idea that a dental surgery is not a place in which to give full vent to one's emotional feelings.

Summary and Conclusion

In this chapter, we have made a distinction between pain as a sensation, pain as the interpretation of that sensation, and pain as the expression and reaction to that interpretation. The magnitude of pain experienced is only partially a function of tissue damage. Other contextual and social variables interact with tissue damage to define and label a sensation as painful and to determine the magnitude of that suffering. The amount of pain expressed is independent of the amount of pain experienced in the sense that the magnitude of experienced pain is not necessarily correlated with the emotional expression of suffering. The main problem in the dental surgery is in the domain of the expression of pain because it is at this level that therapeutic procedures are either facilitated by a stoic response, or hampered by an anti-stoic one. The evidence suggests that the quality of the dentist-patient relationship affects both the perception and the expression of pain.

Pain is an internal, private, and often ambiguous sensation. As Festinger (1954) has shown in his theory of social comparisons, when individuals are faced with ambiguous situations, they turn to their social environment for guidance in how to interpret these situations and how to respond appropriately (e.g., Lambert, Libman, and Poser, 1960). In the case of dental pain, patients ask themselves questions such as: Should it hurt? Do I have to grin and bear it? Can I ask the dentist to stop? Is it permissible to wince, groan, or cry out? Patients are in the surgery by themselves and cannot directly observe how other patients would react in similar circumstances. Consequently, they derive their cues from the overall physical and social context of the surgery, from folklore and the media, and from how they assume other persons like themselves, or persons whom they admire, would respond. For most patients the dental surgery is an unfamiliar and bewildering place. An educational program based on the principle of making the dental surgery a less ambiguous setting should be effective in reducing the pain response by providing patients with guidelines about what they can expect, what their sensations mean, and what is the appropriate response to these sensations. However, such a program will be effective only when there is a good relationship between the dentist and the patient, and the information is presented in a skillful and sensitive manner. Later in this book we shall present a more detailed treatment of the principles of sound patient management.

Part II
Theoretic Models and Their Practical Implications

4
Psychoanalysis and Patient Management

The controversy in general psychology between the behaviorists and the psychoanalysts is reflected in the field of dental psychology. It is apparent from the literature that many dentists, as well as social scientists working in the dental area, have been influenced by the writings of Freud and his followers. In this chapter, the basic elements of the Freudian world view will be presented, and then related to the particular topic of dental anxiety. Following this, a sampling of the literature utilizing the psychoanalytic framework will be critically reviewed.

Freud's Theory of Personality Development

Psychologic explanations of behavior differ according to whether they emphasize contemporary or historical influences in the determination of what people do and how they feel. Behaviorists, as indicated in Chapter 5, assume that *contemporary* events presently surrounding the individual shape that person's thoughts, feelings, and actions, particularly those contemporary environmental forces that mediate reward or punishment for the individual. The Freudians take an entirely different view of the matter. They assume that *past* events, in particular those experiences occurring in the first four or five years of life, determine the adult personality, and that subsequently, contemporary events have very little impact on the basic psychologic core of the person. The two models have clearly different implications for the management of personality change. Whereas the behaviorists set out to modify the contemporary contingencies under which people function, the analysts try to change the individual's perceptions and interpretations of significant events in their past.

A core aspect of Freudian theory is its *developmental* framework. The assumption is that as infants mature, they proceed through clearly defined stages, and that the passage of each phase leaves behind an indelible mark on the personality of the emerging individual. Another central feature of the model is the belief that human nature is essentially hedonic. According to the Freudians, the infant is born with one major tendency, the desire to maximize pleasure and avoid pain. This has been called the *pleasure principle*, and is characterized by the infant's need for immediate (as distinct from delayed) gratification. For example, when young infants are hungry, they cannot wait, but must be fed immediately.

Freud also believed that all pleasure has an erotic component, leading to his much misunderstood theory of *infantile sexuality*. What he meant was that in so far as infants pursue pleasure, they must be regarded as sexually active, which is sometimes misrepresented as implying intercourse, an obviously absurd notion. The theory localizes the pursuit of pleasure in three major areas of the body, the oral, anal, and genital regions. Freud called these the three erogeneous zones because of their capacity to provide pleasure when stimulated. Furthermore, he asserted that there is a developmental sequence during which the various zones come into prominence, corresponding with the major stages of personality development.

The earliest zone to dominate the infant's behavior is the *oral* zone. Consequently, the first stage of personality development is the oral stage. During this phase, the infant's main activity is to suck the breast and later the bottle, not merely for the purpose of ingesting food, but because of the intrinsically pleasurable sensations associated with the act of sucking. For example, when tired or in pain the infant will soothe itself by sucking its thumb. The other important function of the mouth at this stage of life, according to Freud, is to explore the world with it. Small infants are likely to place all objects they encounter, edible or not, in their mouths as a way of getting to know these objects.

The second stage of development is the *anal* stage. During this period a child discovers the possibility of obtaining pleasurable sensations from anal activities. The third stage is the *genital* phase, during which children become aware of their genitals and the immense potential of these organs for pleasure. Masturbation of one form or another is not exclusively a postpubertal phenomenon, but is practiced by most children of preschool age.

Although the child is a hedonic creature, it does not live in a social vacuum. The peopled environment can either facilitate or hinder the achievement of pleasure. For example, childrens' oral needs may be gratified or frustrated depending on the capacity of the mother's breasts, whether children are allowed to suck their thumbs, and on many other circumstances. Anal activity, likewise, is socially constrained, depending as it does on the toilet training philosophy of the parents. Genital activity in children, at least in Western culture, is almost certainly going to be severely curtailed by parents viewing any genital play as unnatural and "dirty." These confrontations between the developing child and its social environment are assumed to have far reaching consequences. According to Freud the adult personality is formed by the way in which various conflicts and situations are resolved when they first arise. This is the notion of *fixation*, or the assumption that current behavior constitutes a replaying of earlier scenes, in the sense that the manner in which some critical oral, anal, or genital crisis was resolved in childhood will set the pattern for the resolution of analogous problems in later life.

For example, the Freudian literature contains assertions that persons fixated at the oral passive stage, will as adults lack drive, be dependent, and find activities such as kissing, smoking, chewing, and eating extremely pleasurable. Oral aggressive persons are supposed to use "biting language," make "cutting remarks," and get pleasure from inflicting pain on others, all activities analogous to having a vigorous attitude toward the breast as babies. The anal stage is deemed to be important because toilet training is the first real crisis in the life of an infant. It is usually the first time that a child seriously encounters social rules and regulations. Toilet training can vary from being very severe to being very lenient—from having too much attention placed on it by the parents to giving it little emphasis. Anal traits, like oral ones fall into two categories defining the end of a continuum. Severe toilet training, according to Freud, can lead in adulthood to an obsession with cleanliness and order, or, if the child rebels against parental control, to excessive sloppiness and carelessness.

Another aspect of the anal stage is that the child discovers that it can please and hence manipulate its mother by using the toilet rather than soiling its clothes. This is the first instance of a social contract in which the child in effect is saying to its mother: "You give me (love) and I will give you a 'present' in the potty. If you don't give me what I want, I will not do it." According to how this childhood scenario is played out, adults can, says Freud, become either excessively retentive, miserly, reluctant to let go, or excessively generous, spendthrift, pouring it all out. Collectors (of stamps, coins, whatever) are supposed to illustrate the anal retentive personality, and what used to be called "Bohemianism" and more recently the "flower children" movement, are illustrative of personalities more interested in expression and distribution than retention.

Freud was an exponent of the golden mean. He believed that healthy adult personalities depended, literally, on the balanced overcoming of various obstacles. Successful child rearing consists of taking a middle ground—it should be neither too severe nor too lax. The main crises, such as weaning, toilet training, and the controlling of the libidinous impulses, should be approached in a balanced manner, in order to produce adult personalities whose oral, anal, and genital traits likewise occupy the middle ground. A special crisis that most children encounter is the triangular relationship between themselves and their two parents. Freud called this the *Oedipus Complex* when it involves a boy, and the *Electra Complex* when it concerns a girl.

The Oedipus situation is difficult for the male child because of the assumption that little boys are sexually attracted to their mothers and therefore come to regard the father as a rival. At the same time, there are strong pressures on a boy to love and respect his father. The son resolves this problem by repressing his sexual love for the mother. Having relinquished his mother as a sex object, the boy ceases to regard his father as a rival, and can now accord him the necessary filial devotion. The next step is for the boy to identify with his father, by which Freud meant that the boy will strive to become like the person whom his mother loves—the person who is in possession of the object that he himself had to reluctantly relinquish. The *Electra Complex* is the mirror image of the Oedipus Complex, the girl child relinquishing her father as a sex object and identifying with her mother.

The Concept of Repression

Freud used the Oedipus and Electra complexes to explain sex-role orientation, which the child presumably acquires through the process of identifying with the parent of the same sex. Implied also in the theory is the notion that an unresolved Oedipus or Electra complex leads to disturbed, weakened, or reversed sex roles, and to ambivalence and vacillation, especially towards authority figures. The Oedipus complex also introduces the concept of repression, which states that unacceptable thoughts and impulses (e.g., incest with one's mother) tend to be banished from consciousness. However, such thoughts do not disintegrate or disappear, because according to Freud, psychic energy cannot be destroyed, only modified. Unacceptable impulses are merely pushed below the level of conscious awareness, where they continue to exist in their original form.

Impulses that have been repressed may be triggered by various circumstances, giving rise to anxiety. The psyche responds by censoring these impulses, pushing them down again, and/or by allowing some of the energy to be dissipated in a disguised or indirect form. For example, dreams and slips of the tongue are supposed to provide an avenue for the expression of unacceptable impulses, and activities such as film going, the theater, literature, and the visual arts can provide vicarious, substitute, or fantasy expression of impulses repugnant to the conscious personality but fascinating to the unconscious mind.

To account for the interaction between the various levels of consciousness, Freud developed a structural model of the mind, containing three main components: the Id, Ego, and Super Ego. The *Id* consists of the primitive urges that we are born with, the survival forces that are energized by powerful erotic and aggressive impulses. The Id operates according to the *pleasure principle*, seeking immediate gratification of its needs regardless of the consequences. However, as the child matures, it begins to realize that in order to fit into society, it has to curb these instinctive drives. In particular, the child discovers that to get maximum pleasure in the long run, it has to be able to tolerate some tension in the short term, to learn to postpone immediate gratification. These are the beginnings of the Self or *Ego*, which as it develops has the function of monitoring the child's commerce with its physical and social environment, and delaying immediate gratification in acordance with the *reality* principle. Finally, as the standards and values of society are inculcated in the child, it develops a conscience or *Super Ego*, which acts as an internalized parent to self-regulate behavior.

The Defense Mechanisms

According to Freud, a good deal of mental effort is exerted by the Ego to prevent Id tendencies from breaking through into consciousness. Freud called these strategies the defense mechanisms. Some of the more frequently mentioned ones include *projection*, or the attribution of the unsavory desire to others; *rationalization*, or the finding of good reasons for bad actions; *overcompensation*, or overemphasizing the opposite of the repressed tendency; and *sublimation*, or the finding of a socially acceptable outlet for the tendency.

In summary, the infant is born a hedonic creature. To live in society the child cannot satisfy every impulse the moment it arises. Socialization consists of learning to postpone, control, and modify the Id impulses. Personality is formed through the interaction between the child's primitive biologic pleasure-seeking needs and the curbing and socializing processes that have been brought to bear on the child in the first four or five years of life. If the restrictions and sanctions imposed on the child are either too severe or too lax, these extremes will be reflected in the adult personality.

Current, contemporary behavior is never taken at face value by psychoanalysts. Two sets of forces are assumed to be operating to distort the behavior, unbeknownst to the actor as well as to the observer. The first is *transference*, or the notion that the manner and style in which a person reacts to a contemporary situation will be determined by the manner in which the person related to the prototype of that situation in childhood. The second is the notion of *unconscious psychic defense*, or the assumption that many situations trigger dormant, repressed impulses. When this occurs, the person feels anxious and reduces the anxiety by resorting to one of the defense mechanisms. The fundamental implication of the psychoanalytic model is that even everyday, "ordinary" behavior contains a large irrational component, in the sense that persons are not fully aware of the reasons for their actions, the purposes that their actions serve, or the nature and extent of the pleasure that they experience.

The Freudian model of mind has been immensely influential in many spheres, not just in psychology. The cinema, theater, literature, visual arts, politics, ethics, and esthetics are only some of the fields that have been affected. In psychology, psychoanalysis has been a dominant force, particularly in the first half of this century. However, since the 1950s, with the development of increasingly sophisticated experimental procedures in the behavioral sciences, there has been a gradual turning away from Freud (Garfield, 1981). Today, the psychoanalytic theory of mind plays a very minor role in the training and curriculum of most psychology students. The reason is that so far, no one has been able to propose a satisfactory method for either confirming or disconfirming the theory, causing many observers to conclude that the model is inherently impervious to empiric scrutiny. As Wolpe (1981) has written, ". . . not a single one of the theory's main propositions has ever been supported by scientifically acceptable evidence" (p. 160). In the absence of empiric proof, contemporary psychology tends to either ignore or reject psychoanalysis, the reaction varying from regarding it as a lot of mumbo jumbo to viewing it as an interesting idea awaiting confirmation. For instance, with respect to the concept of orality, which is of special relevance to the psychology of dentistry, Sandler and Dare (1970) after a comprehensive survey of the literature have concluded ". . . that great care is to be used before ascribing later manifestations (be they character traits or symptoms) to the simple repetition, in later life, of the experiences and attitudes of the infant, and his relations to his biological objects (in particular the mother), during his first months of life, during the so-called oral phase of psychosexual development" (p. 221).

Many social scientists would agree with Salter (1949) that "It is high time that psychoanalysis, like the elephant of fable, dragged itself off to some distant jungle graveyard and died. Psychoanalysis has outlived its usefulness. Its methods are vague, its treatment is long drawn out, and more often than not, its results are insipid and unimpressive" (Salter, 1949, p. 1). Such comments, however, have not deterred many psychoanalysts from continuing their work, nor has there been any noticeable decline in the number of articles and books devoted to expounding the Freudian and neo-Freudian points of view. After all, it is easy for the Freudians to explain their critics' stance by labeling it as transference behavior, and implying that the resistance to psychoanalysis indicates some unresolved childhood crisis.

Despite its poor empiric showing, quite a few social scientists and dentists have used the psychoanalytic model to explicate the relationship between the dentist and the patient. In a way, this is not surprising, as the dental situation has many of the ingredients that Freudians emphasize. The dentist is an authority figure and therefore can be thought of as arousing Oedipal fantasies; dentistry involves the mouth, and this invokes fixations from the oral stage; and body contact between the dentist and the patient may bring about sexually charged tensions and anxieties. In the next section, a representative sample of psychoanalytically oriented studies of the dentist-patient relationship will be reviewed. This will be followed by a critique of the contribution of psychoanalysis to the psychology of dentistry.

Studies of Dental Anxiety Based on Psychoanalytic Principles

Unlike the work influenced by learning theory, which as we shall see in Chapter 5 is primarily concerned with the empiric evaluation of various anxiety reducing techniques, the psychoanalytic literature is highly impressionistic. A good example of the genre is Todes' (1972) paper, titled "The child and the dentist: A psychoanalytic view." The article refers to the oral, anal, and genital phases, and their supposed relationship to the practice of dentistry. Todes writes that whereas to the dentist the oral cavity looks small, to the patient it appears huge; that numbness as a result of a local anesthetic produces a distorted body image; that as a body opening, the mouth is invested with fears of penetration; that patients, particularly children, unconsciously associate dental procedures with masturbation, castration, and other sexual anxieties so that interventions in the mouth inevitably harbor sexual and aggressive overtones; that a child may refuse to open its mouth because it expects to be mutilated by the dentist—a parental figure—for having been naughty; that adolescents, uncertain of their sexual orientation, find their passivity, and the dominance of the dentist particularly disturbing, as the situation, according to Todes (1972) evokes homosexual fantasies and fears. However, no empiric evidence to support these contentions is provided. Todes concludes, as do most of the other writers in this school, that a dentist who understands the psychoanalytic basis of dental aversion will be in a better position to manage the anxious patient. This is a highly debatable conclusion, which will be examined at the end of this review.

Most of the articles in this area cover the same ground, and will therefore only be given brief mention unless the author makes some new point. Martin (1965) and Kirsch (1974) liken the mouth to a cave symbolizing the vagina, and the teeth symbolizing sexual attractiveness, potency, and the penis. Kirsch presents case studies in which patients associated missing teeth with feelings of diminished potency and sexual attractiveness, but one or two such instances hardly constitute empiric evidence for the generality of the relationship.

Sword (1970) poses the often asked questions: Why do patients neglect their teeth, regularly appearing at their six-month appointment with recurrent decay, extensive calculus and debris, and dentures covered with deposits? Why do patients invest considerable time and money in dental treatment and then ignore the instructions about home care that would give them better oral health as well as protecting their investment? As we saw in Chapter 2, the conventional answers include patient ignorance, lack of skill in dental hygiene, placing a low value on oral health, and that because decaying teeth do not necessarily cause pain, patients have no cues to remind them that their oral health is deteriorating and hence are not moved to take appropriate action. Sword, however, offers yet another explanation, grounded in the psychoanalytic dual instinct theory. Freud proposed the existence of two opposing forces, "libido" or the life instinct, and the death instinct. The life instinct is said to energize human creativity, self-preservation, and procreation. The death instinct is said to provide the energy for and "explain" acts of self-destruction, manifested overtly in suicide and more subtly in depressive reactions, fear of success, accident-proneness, self-blame, self-punishment, and so forth. Normally, according to Freud, the two forces function in such a way that the constructive drive is dominant, and the individual can grow and flourish. However, in some psychologically ill persons, self-hate and the tendency to punish or destroy oneself escape from the controlling influence of the libido, and such people contribute actively to their own downfall, either consciously or unconsciously. For example, the Freudian theory of depression states that when people harbor strongly felt but socially unacceptable impulses, such as aggression towards parents or parental figures, the guilt that this arouses is unconsciously relieved by making a sacrifice, usually by turning the destructive drive back on the self. The theory asserts that this can occur quite unconsciously, so that the person is not aware of the hatred felt, will deny such feelings if they are suggested to the patient, and presumably explains why many depressed patients are unable to give a clear reason for their lack of self-esteem.

Sword (1970) extended this theory to account for the phenomenon of oral neglect. Sword states that depressed patients, expiating their unconscious guilt, make a partial sacrifice by neglecting their teeth, implying that the depression must be treated before something can be done about the neglect. Unfortunately, Sword presents no evidence for the assumed link between oral neglect, depression, and self-destruction.

Martin (1965) suggests that the helplessness and passivity that many patients feel arouses homosexual fears in them, that patient often see the dentist in the role of a sadistic attacker and mutilator. These conclusions were drawn after interpreting the responses of dental patients interviewed about their feelings and experience. For example, statements such as "The dentist massacred my teeth," and "If you've got your mouth open, you've got no defense whatsoever," were presented as evidence for the role of the dentist as aggressor. However, it should be obvious that alternate interpretations of such statements are possible.

The Psychoanalytic View of the Dental Profession

The dentists themselves have not escaped the scrutiny of the psychoanalysts. For example, Raginsky (1968) suggests that the professional manner is a defense mechanism masking personal insecurity, apprehension and prejudice; that dentists harbor guilt feelings and unconscious hostility toward some of their patients; that dentists often crave to be needed, loved, and respected, needs that are not always satisfied; and that some emotionally immature dentists displace their personal problems onto their patients.

Raginsky concludes that dentists must have insight into their own personalities in order to become more effective practitioners. However, no evidence is presented regarding the existence and incidence of these neurotic symptoms among dentists.

Martin (1965) states that the profession of dentistry inevitably involves inflicting pain and discomfort on other people. Dentists spend a lot of time in close physical contact with their patients, in a tense relationship that is quite stressful for the dentist. Some dentists, according to Martin, use the dental situation to gratify their own infantile oral and sadistic impulses. Others react to patient hostility by displacing their aggression, notably through antagonism toward the medical profession and dental mechanics. Some defend against their anxieties by withdrawing from personal involvement with their patients, do not work with children, refrain from providing dental hygiene education, and exaggerate an interest in technical competence. These conclusions are based on interviews with and observations of dentists by Martin's research team. However, a nonpsychoanalytically oriented social scientist might arrive at a different set of interpretations.

The Psychoanalytic Typology of Dental Patients

In some branches of psychiatry it is the practice to classify both normal and abnormal individuals according to their personality type. The basis for the classification is often derived from psychoanalytic theory. Some writers have used such personality taxonomies to explain the behavior of dental patients, and then offer advice to dentists on how to manage different personality types. For example, Tarachow (1946) distinguishes between narcissists, compulsives, hysterics, and masochists.

Narcissists are vain, egocentric, need approval and praise, and are mistrustful and suspicious. According to Tarachow, to gain the confidence of such individuals the dentists should be as narcissistic about their work as the patients are about their beauty.

Compulsives are rigid, orderly, and adhere to fixed patterns and schedules. They may be very moralistic, stubborn and unyielding, change their minds with difficulty, and cooperate poorly with others in joint tasks. They may be preoccupied with cleanliness, and they tend to intellectualize experiences and emotions. The dentist, says Tarachow, can establish a working relationship with obsessive patients by appealing (pandering?) to their values of order, cleanliness, and intellect.

Hysterics, according to Tarachow, interpret every experience as a sexual encounter. Hysterics struggle with sexual symbols wherever they go. An elevator moving in a shaft, a train in a tunnel, opening a door, these and a myriad other happenings are constant reminders of sex. Visiting the dentist is treated as a potential seduction. Hysterics are always anxious about sexual temptations and possibilities of rape. Hysterical symptoms include paralyses of various limbs and sensory disturbances such as blindness, deafness, and even toothache that have no somatic base. Tarachow's advice to dentists dealing with hysterics is not to encourage the patient's romantic fantasies, while at the same time recognizing the existence of these feelings and making due allowances for them.

Masochists assume blame and guilt, feel inferior, are unaggressive, tend to agree with others, and lack ambition. According to Tarachow, dentists will find that such patients respond readily to an appeal directed at their sense of obligation, conformity, and duty. Masochists, because of their need to suffer, may even be attracted to painful procedures, making them extremely cooperative dental patients.

An overlapping list of personality types is offered by Friend (1953). However, Friend's advice to dentists is not always identical with Tarachow's. For example, Friend believes that obsessive-compulsives make ideal dental patients because they should conscientiously follow the dentist's instructions about oral hygiene, be punctual, and pay their bills promptly. Dentists should not be too warm, reassuring, or personal with compulsives, but establish a tactful and formal relationship with them.

Types mentioned by Friend that do not appear in the earlier list include the *hypochondriac, homosexual,* and *infantile* patient respectively. Despite the obvious nuisance value of hypochondriacs, Friend counsels patience and tolerance. Active homosexuals, according to Friend, are extremely intolerant of frustration and pain, whereas passive homosexuals may wish to be treated roughly, and it is likely that they will enjoy the dental procedures in a masochistic way, making them ideal patients. Many patients, says Friend, are infantile in some respect, overtly dependent on authority, and lack initiative. Such people also make good (docile?) patients. Finally, both Tarachow and Friend include the *borderline psychotic* type in their classification. This label is attached to people who in the view of some experts are actually insane, but who are able to hide their illness from the lay person and manage to pursue their occupations undetected. According to Friend, 30% of dental patients fit into this category, and, according to him, make as good patients as any other despite their oddities. Friend's advice is to humor such patients but not get involved in their personal problems, delusions, and fantasies.

The reader will recognize in the various personality *types* the oral, anal oedipal *traits* that were said to characterize the oral, anal, and genital *stages* of development. One of the attractions of the psychoanalytic model is its internal consistency. At the same time, this very consistency constitutes a major hazard for the theory as the whole system must either stand or fall together. It is very difficult to partially agree with the model, unlike one's potential attitude to the proverbial curate's egg. Because the various elements of the psychoanalytic system are so interrelated, one must either accept the lot or reject the lot.

Personality Types, Personality Traits, and Situational Demands

With respect to the particular issue of personality types, their existence and utility has been the subject of a good deal of controversy in recent years. Two major criticisms have achieved wide currency and acceptance. The first is that very few individuals fit into a pure type or category (Cattell, 1965). Thus, to be able to accommodate the majority of human kind, and not just the relatively few individuals who happen to be prototypic, would necessitate constructing a taxonomy with a huge number of categories in it. In effect, such taxonomies would become continous scales or dimensions along which individuals would order themselves. Despite the claims of writers such as Tarachow and Friend, only a minority of dental patients, or for that matter psychiatric patients, would fit with any degree of ease into the rather simplistic set of categories generated by the Freudian model. Most individuals behave more or less narcissistically, compulsively, hysterically, or childishly depending on the particular circumstances they find themselves in. This leads to the second point of criticism, directed at the existence and utility of the personality trait concept.

A great deal of recent work has shown that personality traits are not the sole or even primary determinants of behavior (Mischel, 1968). The way that a person acts in a particular situation will depend on two factors: the individual's personality, that being the traits, habits, inclination, propensities, and other permanent characteristics of the person, *and* on the demands of the situation. The response therefore is always the outcome of an interaction between the personal characteristics of the actor and the social situation that provides what has been called the behavioral setting for the act (Barker, 1968, 1979). The relative contribution of the person and the setting to the equation also differs, depending on a variety of conditions. In highly circumscribed situations such as the dental surgery, personality factors should be theoretically less important than the demands of the setting in controlling the behavior of individuals.

The intensity with which the situation can influence the behavior of those caught up in it has been convincingly demonstrated in a series of experiments utilizing a simulated prison. At Stanford University in California (Haney, Banks, and Zimbardo, 1973), and at the University of New South Wales in Sydney (Lovibond, Mithiran, and Adams, 1979), the basements of the psychology department buildings were converted into "jails." Volunteer subjects played the role of either prisoners or guards, the prisoners living in the jail for the duration of the experiment, and the guards commuting to it for their "work shifts." Staff members of the psychology departments acted as the prison superintendent, parole officers, prison chaplain, board of governors, and so forth. The experiments ran for several days, with striking results. The "guards"very quickly began to exhibit traits consistent with their role: they became authoritarian, overbearing, aggressive, and punitive. The "prisoners" likewise behaved appropriately: they became passive, dependent, ingratiating, and devious. And the "prison superintendent" found himself, to his surprise, behaving as a prison administrator and not as a social science researcher.

The volunteers in the experiments were all carefully screened for psychiatric symptoms prior to the commencement of the study. The subjects were randomly assigned to the "guard" or "prisoner" conditions. All subjects were told that they could drop out of the experiment at any time they wished. Nevertheless, most subjects remained in the study till it was terminated, and for the vast majority of the participants the situational pull was so great as to modify their behavior in the direction required by the behavior setting. It should also be noted that much of this behavior could be described as neurotic or even borderline psychotic.

Studies such as the simulated prison experiments cast serious doubt on the premise that behavior is primarily the overt manifestation of basic personality traits, whether established in the first few years of life or conceptualized as a continuously developing set of inner characteristics. The implications for the management of dental anxiety are that dentist who interpret the behavior of their patients purely in terms of the assumed inner characteristics these people are supposedly bringing with them to the surgery, may be insensitive to some of the major sources of dental stress. In particular, such dentists are likely to ignore or deny that the behavior setting of the surgery, and their own role performance in that context can have a significant impact on patient anxiety.

There is another and more specific sense in which the dentist's assumptions about human nature bear directly on the management of dental problems. Freudian psychology regards all overt manifestations as symptoms of some underlying conflict in the psyche of the individual. This hypothesis, for example, has important consequences for thumb sucking and its treatment, and the issue has generated quite a large literature (see Ayer and Gale, 1970, for a review). Psychoanalytic theory maintains that thumb sucking is instinctive and therefore normal in infancy, since it gratifies the oral needs of the young child. However, in later life thumb sucking is deemed to be indicative of some underlying emotional problem. The psychoanalytic view considers it pointless to treat just the symptom, which in this case might involve discouraging children from sucking their thumbs by punishing them for the act, or preventing them from placing their thumbs in the mouth by requiring the patient to wear mittens. Such interventions would not be favored by psychoanalytically oriented dentists, because of the assumption that the treatment would not reach the real, deep-seated cause of the disturbance. Indeed, the dentist would actively reject such a therapy, because the Freudian theory of symptom substitution holds that if a symptom is suppressed, it will simply appear in another form. In the present case the theory implies that if a child is prevented from sucking its thumb, it may turn to compulsive mas-turbation, temper tantrums, or other behavior disorders as a means of ex-pressing the underlying unconscious conflict. Dentists who accept this view will refrain from taking any direct action with thumb-sucking patients, other than to suggest that the patient seeks psychiatric treatment. This advice will be based on the assumption that nothing can be done about the symptom until the underlying cause is treated, and if the behavior is restricted it will simply reappear in another guise.

It is interesting to contrast the learning theory account of thumb sucking with the above view. Learning theory regards thumb sucking as an acquired response, not necessarily serving any underlying functions. The genesis of thumb sucking is deemed to be similar to the origin of any other habit. It is assumed that initially the thumb or finger come into contact accidentally with the mouth and are sucked. The sucking is gratifying because it is analo-gous to feeding, so the child repeats the behavior. In the process, the child acquires a habit that is pleasurable but also detrimental to oral health. If this is the correct interpretation of thumb sucking then there is no reason why the habit should not be unlearned, using reward and punishment as the means of extinguishing the behavior. Nor should the dentist be worried about the symptom appearing in another guise, as a review of the literature by Yates (1958) concluded that symptom substitution theory has not been supported by any empiric evidence. Indeed, Ayer and Gale (1970) describe several stu-dies that have successfully used behavior modification techniques to reduce thumb sucking, without producing any unfavorable consequences such as creating new symptoms or problems. This was confirmed by Cerny (1981) in a study of 600 Australian children, where it was found that 109 or only 18% were digit suckers. (Of these 87 or 80% sucked their thumb, and 22 [20%] sucked a finger.) Cerny reports that the majority of the digit suckers gave up their habit spontaneously or gradually without any assistance other than occasional parental encouragement, and only 18 children (or 17%) showed some palatal distortion as a consequence of their sucking habit. Those chil-dren treated for sucking by a doctor or dentist responded to the treatment, and the sucking was not replaced by any substitute habits or emotional prob-lems.

In an American study, Cipes, Miraglia, and Gaulin-Kremer (1986) used the techniques of monitoring and contingency contracting to treat eleven children aged 5 to 9 who were persistent thumb suckers. Monitoring involves keeping a record of the desired behavior (in this instance refraining from thumb sucking) and rewarding it. Contingeny contracting consists of a for-mal agreement between the parent and the child in which a behavioral goal is set for the child and a reward for achieving that goal is agreed on. When the child meets the goal, he or she is rewarded by the parent according to the agreement. If the goal is not achieved, the child is not rewarded (nor is it punished). In the present study, parents monitored the behavior of their children during set periods, eight times daily. Absence of thumb sucking was recorded at each observation by placing stars on a printed calendar that was displayed in a conspicuous place. The children were given feedback, praise and a star for not sucking their thumb, and no star or praise if thumb sucking occurred during the period. Some of the parents also set up contingency contracts for reaching a jointly agreed upon goal. The results showed that thumb sucking declined notably from a preintervention baseline, and this reduction persisted for the six months during which the study was conducted.

Dentists other than those working within the Freudian framework will tend to reject the symptom substitution hypothesis. Whether they accept learning theory or not, faced with a thumb-sucking patient, they will at least not be prevented by their beliefs from recommending direct treatment aimed at extinguishing the habit, if that is an important dental therapeutic goal. It follows, therefore, that dentists' beliefs about human nature are not just of academic interest because these ideas intrude directly into the management of the patient's illness. Thumb sucking provides a sharp illustration of how different theories can lead to diametrically opposed management strategies, but is only one example among many. Most if not all management problems are affected in varying degrees by the dentists' assumptions about what makes their patients tick.

Australasian Studies

In Australia and New Zealand, the application of the psychoanalytic model to dentistry has achieved some attention through the work of two influential writers, R.T. Martin and J.P. Walsh. Martin (1965, 1970) is a psychoanalyst, and was commissioned by The Dental Health Education and Research Foundation of the University of Sydney to investigate dentist-patient relationships. This research has been referred to earlier in this chapter and also reviewed in the chapter dealing with surveys. Walsh (1953, 1956, 1959, 1962, 1964, 1965) is a Melbourne-trained physician and dentist, working in Dunedin. Walsh's theme is that many oral symptoms have a psychogenic or psychosomatic basis, including the inability to open the mouth, pain in the face, a swollen face, tender or painful teeth, septic teeth that must come out, dentures that cannot be worn, and bad breath or a bad taste (Walsh, 1953, 1956). The interpretation is psychoanalytic. The inability to open the mouth is diagnosed as hysteric trismus, corresponding to vaginismus; fear of losing teeth is taken to symbolize loss of fertility; patients who insist on having their teeth out are expiating unconscious guilt; and bad breath is a conversion hysteria. In later papers the list of psychogenic symptoms is extended to include clicking jaw and bruxism (Walsh, 1962, 1965), the latter said to be due to the patient's unconscious attempts to prevent the manifestation of aggressive tendencies.

According to Walsh (1959), anxiety, feelings of resentment, guilt, frustration, inadequacy, dependency, lack of security, indecision, loss of love, separation, and aggression can all produce oral symptoms. Walsh (1964) relates patient behavior to the defense mechanisms. Some patients repress their dental fears by becoming indifferent to dental health. Some persons become dentists because they had an unpleasant dental experience as a child and in order to overcome their anxieties, identify with the aggressor. Some patients overcompensate by denying their fear, displace or disguise their anger at the dentist through humor, and develop oral symptoms as a substitute for the gratification of blocked needs, or to punish themselves. However, only a few case studies are presented by Walsh to substantiate his assertions, and every one of the cases could be explained without reference to the principle of unconscious motivation.

Conclusion

Many writers, both dentists and social scientists, have extended the principles of psychoanalysis to the dental surgery. However, the usefulness of such an extension can be questioned because there is very little evidence either for or against the psychoanalytic theory of dental aversion in particular, and the behavior of dental patients in general. The following list summarizes the main weaknesses of the psychoanalytic account of dental behaviour:

1) The central assumptions of the psychoanalytic model of the mind are not capable of being tested empirically (Wolpe, 1981). A requirement of the scientific method is that the phenomenon under scrutiny can be publicly observed and reproduced by independent investigators (Lin, 1976). Practically all of the phenomena of psychoanalysis consist of the subjective interpretations that individual analysts make of the subjective states of their particular clients.

2) Even if some of the aspects of the Freudian model could be supported empirically, the extension of these ideas to dentistry rests on analogy, and on the subjective interpretations that individual dentists make of the conscious and unconscious states of their patients.

3) The psychoanalytic approach implies that the behavior of dental patients is essentially irrational, that patients are not fully aware of the reasons for their behavior—in effect, nothing is what it seems because patients are acting out infantile fantasies, or employing one or more of the defense mechanisms to cope with unacceptable erotic, aggressive, or self-destructive impulses. Dentists concentrating on the latent content, on what may or may not be below the surface, could miss noticing or not give sufficient emphasis to the manifest content of the patient's complaint—to the overt communications and symptoms being presented by the patient.

4) The psychoanalytic model locates the reasons for the patients' feelings and acts within the personality of the individual. Intrapsychic explanations of behavior provide a very one-sided view because they ignore the contribu-

tion of the situation in determining how people act and what they feel. Dentists who adopt an intrapsychic view will tend to leave out of the equation their own actions, and the impact of the behavior setting. This would be a serious ommission, as research has shown that interpsychic variables known to have an effect on patient behavior include such aspects as the design and layout of the surgery; the demeanor of the other members of the dental treatment team such as nurses, receptionists, and technicians; whether preventive or restorative care is emphasized; policies regarding the presence of relatives during the treatment; financial aspects; and the many other contextual influences that have been discussed elsewhere in this book.

5) Even if the Freudian view of the world were correct, dentists who adopt the psychoanalytic model as the basis for patient management are not provided with a feasible treatment rationale, short of sending all of their patients to be psychoanalyzed. Indeed, because of the theory of symptom substitution, in many instances dentists would be required not to intervene, particularly if the intervention could be interpreted as punitive by the patient. This could lead to some patently absurd consequences, with dentists refusing to treat dental illness on psychiatric grounds. To the extent that the model has any practical implications, these tend to favor the dentist, enabling practitioners to unload any guilt they might feel about inflicting pain or not effecting a cure. For example, the psychoanalytically oriented dentist can blame oral neglect on the self-destructive tendencies of the patient, conveniently ignoring that the most parsimonious explanation for poor oral hygiene is due to many dentists being very bad health educators. In turn, the reason why dentists are not effective health communicators is that by and large they do not receive adequate training in how to teach oral hygiene. Attributing poor oral hygiene to the death instinct is unlikely to improve the dental curriculum to any marked extent, although it can justify the status quo with respect to health education.

What positive aspects can be drawn from the Freudian model of the mind? It is certainly true that people are not always fully aware of their feelings, or correctly interpret their motives. Individuals undoubtedly have a capacity for self-delusion, and like to present themselves in the best possible light (Crowne and Marlow, 1964). However, the majority of people are reasonably in touch with their inner selves. Only a minority exhibit the extremes of tortuous and devious behavior, the heady mixture of manifest and latent content so beloved of psychoanalytic case-study writers. Dentists should certainly be aware that at times a patient of the opposite sex could be lusting after them, that they remind some of their younger patients of their parents, or that some of the patients may be afraid that losing a tooth will diminish their attractiveness. Undoubtedly, a small proportion of dental patients should be visiting a psychiatrist rather than or as well as a dentist, and the psychopathologic ramifications of dental practice should certainly not be dismissed without careful evaluation (Gobetti, 1981). However, most patients do not visit the dentist in order to give expression to their latent, infantile needs. Rather, patients come to the surgery primarily for dental treatment and bring with them fears and anxieties that relate to the here and now, and not to some traumatic event in distant childhood.

Dentists overly steeped in the principles of psychoanalysis may look for and find "explanations" that have no substance from the patients' perspective, or may be regarded as trivial by the patient, thereby decreasing rather than increasing the level of communciation and trust between the dentist and the patient. The minority of patients who are walking case studies will be easy to identify, but it is very doubtful whether anything that the dentist does will have an impact on their behavior. The material presented in this chapter leads to the conclusion that psychoanalysis has very little relevance for the practice of dentistry.

5
Social Learning Theory and Patient Management

The core notion of social learning theory is that behavior is shaped and maintained by its consequences. Two broad principles have dominated the thinking in this area. These are the *law of effect* and the *principle of contiguity*. The law of effect (Thorndike, 1932), also known as instrumental or operant conditioning (Skinner, 1953), states that responses that are rewarded (reinforced) (Hull, 1951) will persist and increase in frequency, whereas actions that are punished or have aversive consequences, will decrease in frequency and ultimately be extinguished (disappear) from the response repertoire of the individual. The principle of contiguity (Guthrie, 1952), also referred to as classic conditioning (Pavlov, 1927), states that two responses will become associated with each other, regardless of content or effect, simply if they are temporally contiguous, that is, if they are presented to the individual in close succession. This kind of learning is known as Pavlovian conditioning, so called after the Russian physiologist who introduced the idea into the literature. Pavlov was studying the secretion of saliva in dogs. His method was to place different morsels of food into the dogs' mouths and measure the resulting flow of saliva. He noticed that after a while the dogs began to salivate at the sight of the food, the container, and even the white coat of the laboratory attendant. In other words, the dogs had learned to associate these items with the administration of the food into their mouths.

Literally hundreds of thousands of experiments have been conducted using practically every living creature and most of their habits, to confirm and elaborate the principles of learning theory. In the case of human beings, studies of the acquisition of conditioned responses have ranged from the narrow and specific reflex of the eye blink (Beecroft, 1966), to the general learning of one's culture (Guthrie, 1975).

Fear

Fear is a response of the organism to real or imagined threat. In human beings, most fears are learned rather than innate responses, an issue that we will return to later. Traditionally, fear in human beings has been measured in three ways: a) through self-report—by asking persons to indicate, on a suitable scale, how afraid they feel, b) by observing persons in the vicinity of feared objects and inferring the extent of their fear from their overt behavior, such as trembling, facial muscle tension, or approach-avoidance patterns, and c) by recording changes in various physiologic processes such as heart rate and skin conductance, generally assumed to mediate the psychologic experience of fear.

From the above it can be seen that the fear reaction is assumed to have a connative, behavioral, and physiologic component. Empirically, however, the three categories of measures do not correlate very highly with each other (Hodgson and Rachman, 1974; Rachman and Hodgson, 1974). This may be due to measurement error or because other factors such as level of arousal affect the covariation between the various components, or because the three-components assumption is in error. Whatever the explanation, this problem is only one of the many complexities in this area that tend to be glossed over.

Fear Conditioning

Learning theory assumes that fear has the same logical properties as any other response, that it is learned, and that its acquisition follows the general principles of learning. This is contrary to the popular belief that people are innately afraid of dangerous situations. With the possible exception of loud noises, to which babies react instinctively with a startle response (Gibson and Walk, 1960; Goodenough and Tyler, 1959), behaviorists assert that individuals learn their fears in the sense that certain situations, including quite innocuous ones, acquire the property of evoking fear and anxiety for that person. The experiment introducing this idea was the classic Watson and Rayner (1920) study, in which Albert, an 11-month-old baby, was taught to fear a white rat. Initially, Albert was quite unafraid of the animal, touching and playing with it. During the experiment, the investigators struck a suspended steel bar with a hammer whenever Albert reached out to touch the rat. In other words, an experimental trial consisted of the rat followed by a loud noise. After seven trials, Albert had developed a fear reaction to the rat. Even without the loud noise, at the sight of the rat Albert would begin to cry and avoid the rat. Albert had become a victim of classic conditioning. To be even handed, it should be noted that this report has been criticized on the same grounds as many of the studies in the psychoanalytic tradition, namely that the conclusions were based on only a single subject and the results were apparently never replicated in their original form (Harris, 1979; Samelson,

1980). Be that as it may, the principle of emotional conditioning had been articulated, and has had a significant influence on subsequent research and theorizing ever since.

The Terminology of Classic Conditioning

The language of classic conditioning contains four key terms: unconditioned stimulus, conditioned stimulus, unconditioned response, and conditioned response. In Albert's case, the unconditioned stimulus was the loud noise that elicited the unconditioned response of fear. The conditioned stimulus was the rat, which was systematically paired with the unconditioned stimulus, the loud noise. Eventually, the conditioned stimulus, the rat, began to elicit the same reaction as the unconditioned stimulus (the noise), namely fear. In other words, fear, which is the unconditioned response to a loud noise, had through temporal juxtaposition become the conditioned response to the rat. It should be remembered that previously Albert had regarded the rat as an emotionally neutral or even mildly pleasant object. But once the rat was associated with the loud noise, it took on the noxious property of that sound. Figure 5.1 presents the classical conditioning paradigm in schematic form.

Classic and Instrumental Conditioning Combined

The next development in the explanation of fear acquisition occurred when the *law of effect* (instrumental conditioning) was combined with the contiguity principle (classic conditioning). This was done by Mowrer (1960a, b), who proposed a two-factor theory of fear and avoidance. The first stage follows the principles of classic conditioning as described in the preceding section, in which previously neutral stimuli acquire, through association, the noxious properties of an inherently aversive stimulus. The second stage involves terminating the conditioned fear (in Albert's case to the white rat) by withdrawing from the source and avoiding its vicinity. Such avoidance behavior is instrumentally reinforcing because it reduces the fear that was aroused by

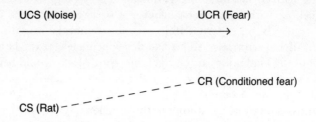

Figure 5.1. The classic conditioning paradigm.

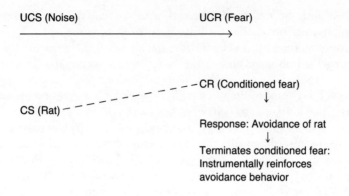

Figure 5.2. Classic and instrumental conditioning paradigms combined to account for fear acquisition and avoidance behavior.

the conditioned stimulus (the rat). Figure 5.2 presents the combined classic and instrumental conditioning paradigms, in schematic form.

Let us briefly recapitulate the argument so far. Individuals and animals develop conditioned fears to previously neutral stimuli because of their association through mere contiguity with some inherently noxious condition. They also discover that they can instrumentally reduce the fear by avoiding the stimulus that has acquired the anxiety-arousing properties. This paradigm was avidly embraced to explain the acquisition of phobias, including dental phobias. The argument goes as follows: At some point in the patient's history the previously neutral dental surgery was paired with pain. If this happened often enough, or if the pain was sufficiently intense, in due course the dental situation would come to elicit fear and anxiety irrespective of whether further actual pain was being experienced. The patients, in order to reduce or eliminate this fear, would avoid taking dental treatment. However, there are several problems with the learning paradigm of phobic fears, casting doubt on whether conditioning can fully account for the phobias, including dental phobia. These problems will now be reviewed.

Extinction

A great many studies have established that conditioned responses wane and finally disappear if the pairings between the conditioned stimulus and the unconditioned stimulus are discontinued, that is, if the conditioned stimulus is repeatedly presented unaccompanied by its usual reinforcer (Kimble, 1961). For example, in the case of Albert, if on subsequent occasions the rat were to have been repeatedly presented without the noise, Albert's fear of the creature should have gradually diminished and finally disappeared. What would have been the consequences of the diminished fear on Albert's behavior toward the rat? It will be remembered that the theory states that escaping from a feared object will have the effect of reducing the fear, and is therefore reinforcing. But once the fear has disappeared, avoiding the object is no longer reinforcing, and so the avoidance behavior, too, should extinguish.

However, contrary to these theoretic expectations, a great many fears and their associated avoidance behaviors persist in real life, in the clinic, and in the laboratory (Bandura, 1977; Clarke and Jackson, 1983; Seligman, 1971), long after the cessation of any pairing with an inherently aversive event. The dental situation provides a good example: Modern dental techniques have greatly reduced the amount of pain associated with most therapeutic procedures. Theoretically, this should gradually extinguish patients' fear and avoidance behaviors. Yet for many patients the dental situation continues to be a source of severe anxiety.

The Equipotentially Premise

A central assumption in learning theory has been that the laws and mechanisms of learning are the same across species, stimuli, and responses. In the context of the present discussion, this assumption has two important consequences. The first is the belief that results obtained in the laboratory using animal subjects can be generalized to human beings in natural settings, including dental patients. The second is the assumption that any stimulus is capable of becoming a conditioned fear stimulus provided that it is paired closely, in time and space, with some aversive event.

Seligman and Hager (1972) have reviewed evidence casting doubt on both of these assumptions. What the data suggests instead is that the degree and kind of conditioning (learning) taking place is in part determined by the intrinsic properties of the conditioned and unconditioned stimulus, and the particular relationship between them. This idea will be expanded on below in the next section, "Preparedness." Seligman and Hager's conclusion, despite its formulation in learning theory terms, is highly consistent with the social-psychologic account of learning, which emphasizes the importance of the relationship between the learner, the material being learned, the source of the learning, and the social context within which the learning occurs. As we shall see later, all these variables have implications for the management of anxiety in the dental surgery.

Preparedness

Seligman (1970, 1971) has proposed that some stimuli, because of their biologic or adaptive significance, are more easily conditioned to produce fear than other, adaptively irrelevant stimuli. Stimuli that readily acquire aver-

sive properties are said to be biologically prepared for their phobic development. Some experimental support for the notion of preparedness does exist.
For example, it is much easier to condition fear using electric shock as the
unconditioned stimulus, to pictures of snakes and spiders than to pictures of
houses, flowers, and mushrooms (Ohman, Eriksson, and Olofsson, 1975;
Ohman, Fredrikson, Hugdahl and Rimmo, 1976). Presumably it is adaptive
to fear snakes and spiders but not flowers and mushrooms. In a recent study
(referred to in Fredrikson and Ohman, 1979), it was found easier to condition phylogenetically fear-relevant stimuli such as snakes or spiders, than to
condition ontogenetically fear-relevant stimuli such as guns, further supporting the biologic notion of preparedness. Relating these ideas to the question
of dental aversion, there is no reason to suppose that dentists should be considered either phylogenetically or ontogenetically prepared to serve as
fear-inducing stimuli because their function is to assist rather than harm
their patients. The evidence supports this view: In an epidemiologic study
of common fears and phobias, Agras, Sylvester, and Oliveau (1969) found
that 390 out of every 1,000 people feared snakes, in comparison to only
198 fearing dentists.

The Traumatic Conditioning Experience

A core assumption of the learning theory account of avoidance acquisition is
that the person should have been exposed to at least one conditioning experience, specifically, that at least one pairing of the conditioned stimulus
with an inherently noxious, unconditioned stimulus should have happened to
the individual. To test this implication, a number of investigators have asked
phobic persons to recall a specific traumatic event that preceded or coin-
cided with the onset of their fear (e.g., Buglass, Clarke, Henderson, Kreitman, and Presley, 1977; Lazarus, 1971; Rimm, Janda, Lancaster, Nahl, and
Dittmar, 1977). These studies indicate that very few people can remember
any occurrence that they would regard as having precipitated their fear. The
actual rate of persons reporting a direct traumatic experience varied from
2% in one study to a maximum of 35% (Rimm et al., 1977), leaving the great
majority of phobics unable to pinpoint such an event. There are exceptions to
this trend. For instance, all 34 of Lautch's (1971) dental phobic subjects
reported having had an unpleasant dental experience in their childhood. But
most people find visiting the dentist relatively unpleasant, so Lautch's results
do not explain why these particular patients developed a phobia whereas
others did not. Hence Lautch's study cannot be used to either confirm or
deny the general view that it is often difficult to identify the specific genesis of
a phobia. It is certainly possible that people may forget or repress their
traumatic experiences. Nevertheless, findings such as these constitute a
major unresolved problem for the learning theory account of fear acquistion.
The studies reviewed above were primarily concerned with establishing

the antecedent conditions to phobic reactions. Studies have also looked at the effect of previous experience on less extreme reactions to dentistry, in particular on dental anxiety. For instance, Rankin and Harris (1984) asked 258 dental patients to fill out a Dental Experience Questionnaire and also administered two dental anxiety scales to them. The results showed that anxiety was related to the patients' previous dental experience, those patients with bad experiences having higher anxiety scores, particularly if the most recent dental experience was negative.

Treatment of Fear Based on Learning Theory Principles

A variety of fear-reducing techniques have been developed, of which the best known are systematic desensitization (Wolpe, 1969), flooding or implosion (Boulougouris and Marks, 1969), and modeling (Bandura, Blanchard, and Ritter, 1969, Bandura, Grusec, and Menlove, 1967). All the techniques depend on exposing the person to the object that is feared, until the fear is desensitized or extinguished, or until the person learns to control the fear. The exposure is usually imaginal in that the subjects are asked to imagine the fear-arousing scene. Under desensitization the exposure is gradual: subjects, while relaxed, imagine increasingly more distressing scenes. Under flooding the exposure is sudden: the subjects are asked to imagine the situation that is the most frightening for them. Under modeling the exposure is vicarious: the afflicted person observes another individual being exposed to the feared situation.

Research regarding the effectiveness of the various techniques consistently shows that relaxation techniques alone (teaching subjects to relax their muscles) are about as effective in reducing fear as techniques depending on imaginal exposure of the feared object (e.g., Borkovec and Sides, 1979; Denney, 1974; Goldfried and Trier, 1974; Kazdin and Wilcoxon, 1976). Although methodologic difficulties undoubtedly play a role in this finding, nevertheless here too there is an unresolved problem for the learning theory account of acquired fears.

Ethical Considerations

Behavior modification, like psychoanalysis, has its critics and there are some social scientists who are vehemently opposed to the method. Unlike the criticism of psychoanalysis, however, the complaint is not that behavior modification techniques are useless, but rather that they work too well, giving excessive power to the therapist and taking too much choice away from the client. An extreme version of this point of view is represented in the following passage, written by two well-known and respected clinicians: "The basis of the behavior modification techniques (deprivation, punishment, terror, exploitation, disgust, bribery) have been with us through the centuries. In civilized communities, however, most of these tactics have long been abandoned by fair-minded, humane individuals. Thus, the behaviorist model, under the cloak of scientific respectability, has not only re-introduced but has encouraged the use of these degrading, destructive, dehumanizing, totalitarian tactics not only in mental hospitals but in prisons, industrial settings and schoolrooms as well" (Braginsky and Braginsky, 1976, p. 76). Nevertheless, despite views such as these, behavior modification is being widely practiced in a variety of contexts, including the management of dental patients (Melamed, 1979).

Studies of Dental Anxiety Based on Learning Theory Principles

Despite some of the unresolved problems inherent in social learning theory, many investigators of dental anxiety have used this framework to guide their research. Some of these studies will now be reviewed. Implicit in many of the investigations is the idea that dental fear is somehow irrational, that it is mildly (or in some cases, severely) phobic in nature. A phobia has been defined as ". . . a special form of fear which (1) is out of proportion to demands of the situation, (2) cannot be explained or reasoned away, (3) is beyond voluntary control, and (4) leads to avoidance of the feared situation" (Marks, 1969, p. 3). Later, evidence will be presented to indicate that the "irrational fear" model of dental anxiety cannot be empirically sustained, and that it paints a misleading picture of the average dental patient. For the moment, however, the literature will be reviewed as it stands.

From a methodologic point of view, many of the studies lack sophistication. Some are little more than impressions and clinical observations, and as such, subject to bias. For instance, Keys, Field, and Korboot (1978) conducted an "experiment" (their term) in which *two* fearful patients were given instructions and praise. No control subjects were employed. Nevertheless, Keys et al. were willing to conclude that instruction and praise combined are effective in facilitating cooperative behavior. Other studies have a polemic rather than empiric bent, the aim of the author being to persuade the profession to adopt a particular course of action. Others are carefully conducted scientific investigations. The studies to be reviewed have been deliberately selected to provide a reflection of what is available. The literature is huge and beyond the scope of this book to cover exhaustively. The examples have been arranged in a rough hierarchy, beginning with impressionistic studies short on rigor, extending to well controlled and sophisticated experiments.

The major practical concern of the writers being reviewed in this section, is the management of anxious patients. Wright and Lange (1976) were particularly interested in developing techniques that would make children more at ease in the surgery. Wright and Lange assumed that dental anxiety is learnt, specifically due to variables such as previous medical and dental experiences;

maternal anxiety towards dental treatment; physical and emotional disability; an unstable home life; and cultural attitudes toward health care. However, the authors present no evidence regarding the incidence of these events in the lives of their patients. Their method for reducing anxiety was to relax the patient either verbally or through training, on the quite reasonable assumption that relaxation reciprocally inhibits anxiety (Wolpe, 1969). They also positively reinforced desirable behavior through attention, interest, and praise; and nonreinforced undesirable behavior by ignoring it. However, again no data regarding the efficacy of these procedures was provided.

Cosgrove (1976) also assumed that dental anxiety develops in childhood as a result of negative experiences, and some means for allaying these fears are proposed. The methods include explanation, a professional manner that will make the patient like the dentist, audio-sedation with white noise or music, relaxation, hypnosis, and pharmaceutical sedation. However, Cosgrove provides no empiric data on the degree to which these various techniques actually reduce dental anxiety.

Hill and O'Mullane (1976) present what amounts to a theoretic cost-benefit analysis of three major methods being used with apprehensive children. The techniques are desensitization, sedation, and general anesthesia. The authors review studies showing that desensitization tends to be more time consuming than either sedation or anesthesia, with seven to nine pretreatment sessions not uncommon. However, there are problems with sedation: oral sedation is unpredictable and intravenous sedation can produce unintended general anesthesia with an increase in dosage. General anesthesia is undesirable because of the complete loss of the protective laryngeal reflexes, and because of the small but real risk of complications. Many authorities also recommend that a specialist anesthetist, using special equipment, should administer the anesthetic, thereby adding to the cost and complexity of the procedure. Hill and O'Mullane propose an alternative method that they call "gradual acclimatization to operative dentistry," that incorporates the aim of preventive care. In effect, the children get used to dental procedures through learning how to care for their teeth. The rationale of the program is carefully explained to the parents, and their cooperation enlisted.

In the first visit, a history is taken, a brief examination made, and the child is praised for coming to see the dentist. The second visit is taken up with toothbrushing instructions and dietary advice. No work as yet is done in the child's mouth. In the third visit, the children are asked to demonstrate their toothbrushing skills, are praised, and at this stage the dentist will take over the brushing, move the child into the chair, and commence simple intraoral procedures. In the fourth session the diet is discussed, fluoride is applied to the child's teeth, and further intraoral procedures are gradually introduced. Unfortunately, the authors provide no quantitative data about the effectiveness of gradual acclimatization in reducing dental anxiety.

Quite a few studies refer to how much time behavior modification techniques consume. However, Weisenberg and Epstein (1973) present a case study in which they used four methods, desensitization, forced exposure, rehearsal, and modeling, respectively, claiming that they were able to reduce the fear of a 2-year-old child at a cost of only three 15-minute appointments. An unusual feature of this case was the rehearsal manipulation, which consisted of giving the parents a plastic mirror and asking them to "play dentist" at home with the patient, praising (i.e., rewarding) the child for appropriate responses.

Gatchel (1980) compared the effectiveness of desensitization against group discussion. Nineteen fearful patients were divided into three sections, two experimental groups and a control group. The experiment subjects met for six sessions, as a *group*. Subjects in the desensitization condition were first given training in relaxation. Then they were instructed to visualize dental scenes in an ascending order of fearfulness. After each session, a group discussion took place, led by a facilitator who encouraged coping attempts. Subjects in the education/discussion condition discussed their past and present experiences of dental anxiety during their six sessions but did not undergo desensitization. The control subjects did not participate in either desensitization or group discussion. The results showed a greater reduction of anxiety as measured by the Corah Dental Anxiety Scale, in the densensitization condition than in the two other groups. On other measures of dental fear the two experiment groups differed significantly from the control group, indicating that both methods have an effect in reducing fear. This study is noteworthy more for its technique than its outcome, in suggesting that behavior modification does not need to be individually administered but can be achieved in a group context, and hence becomes more economic. There is even the suggestion that under some conditions group-administered desensitization may be more effective than when individuals are trained in isolation.

Machen and Johnson (1974) conducted an experiment in which they randomly assigned preschool patients to three groups: a systematic desensitization, model learning, and control condition, respectively. The children in the two experimental conditions visited the surgery one week before their first dental appointment. In the desensitization condition, the children were introduced to the equipment normally used in dental practice. The items were arranged in an ascending order according to their anxiety-inducing properties, beginning with objects such as the mirror, and ending with the chair and the handpiece. In the model learning condition, the children watched a videotape of a child behaving positively during dental treatment, and being verbally reinforced by the dentist. The behavior of all of the children was then rated during three subsequent dental visits. The results showed that on the second and third visits the behavior of the children in the two experimental groups was significantly less negative than that of the children in the control group. There were no differences between any of the groups on the first visit. Finally, the two experimental groups did not differ from each other on any of the visits. This study provides partial empiric support for the efficacy of desensitization and modeling in reducing dental anxiety in children. The results are also consistent with the bulk of the behavior therapy evaluation literature, in not finding any differences between the various forms of treatment.

Corah, Gale, and Illig (1979a) compared the relative efficacy of relaxation and distraction to reduce dental anxiety. The patients were 48 men and 48 women. Subjects were randomly assigned to one of three conditions: a relaxation condition, in which patients listened through earphones to a recorded voice instructing the subjects to relax various muscles; a distraction condition, in which patients played a video ping pong game on a television monitor mounted near the ceiling, with a joy stick clamped to the arm of the dental chair; and a control group. The rather complex results suggest that relaxation was superior to distraction in reducing anxiety, although both methods had a positive effect on the patients. In a second study with the same design, Corah, Gale, and Illig (1979b) added a perceived control condition, in which patients are given a button switch that activates a buzzer and a light; subjects can press this button if they wish the dentist to pause, or if they wish to communicate with the surgeon. Eighty adult patients participated in this study and were randomly assigned to the various conditions. Essentially the same results were obtained as in the previous study: relaxation and distraction, in that order, were effective in alleviating stress. Perceived control had no significant effect on reducing anxiety.

Systematic desensitization can be regarded as an instance of the more general principle of counter-conditioning, where the patient is gradually guided into making responses that are incompatible with an existing undesired response, in this instance, dental anxiety. In an interesting application of this principle, Nevo and Shapira (1986) have proposed that the use of humor might be an effective counter-conditioned response to dental anxiety. They interviewed 10 dentists about their use of humor in managing child patients and whether this reduced anxiety. Many of these dentists reported that they explicitly used humoros statements, jokes, puns, quips, riddles, and rhymes, as a means of countering dental anxiety, on the assumption that humoros feelings and cognitions are incompatible with and should therefore displace anxious ones. The other assumed function of humor is to increase rapport between the dentist and the patient. However, no independent evidence for these outcomes is presented by the authors. As a comment on this approach, provided it is not overdone, a cheerful dentist and surgery is certainly preferable over a gloomy one because at the very least it should contribute to a better dentist-patient relationship. But the dentist must be careful that the humor does not disparage the patient, and that the level of humor matches the mental development and to some extent the mood of the client.

The technique of flooding has also been investigated in a dental context. Unlike systematic desensitization where the stimuli are presented in an ascending order of fearfulness, the flooding technique requires subjects to imagine the most fear-arousing situations they can tolerate. In a study of 50 phobic patients, Mathews and Rezin (1977) found that of those subjects exposed to flooding, 48% successfully completed all necessary dental treatment within the two month follow-up period, in comparison to only 30% of subjects in the control condition, who had been trained to relax but not exposed to flooding.

Not all investigators accept that the different techniques will all produce similar results. Adelson and Goldfried (1970) wanted to establish that modeling reduces dental anxiety more efficiently than desensitization, the "tell, show, do" procedure, or premedication. Two children took part in the study: Amy, who had little dental anxiety, and Penny, for whom the authors anticipated a management problem. Penny watched while Amy was being examined by the dentist. Amy was cheerful, responsive, and cooperative throughout the session and was given a reward as she left. Subsequently Penny was examined, and contrary to what had been anticipated, the treatment proceeded smoothly. The authors attributed this outcome to Penny modeling herself on Amy's behavior. However, it should be noted that this study lacks a control group, in not providing information in how anxious Penny would have acted in the absence of a positive model, or how well she would have behaved if she had been exposed to some other procedure.

White, Akers, Green, and Yates (1974) extended the Adelson and Goldfried study with a more rigorously designed experiment. The subjects were 15 anxious girls between 4 and 8 years of age. The authors manipulated the modeling behavior with the help of an experimental confederate, an 8-year-old girl who underwent simulated treatment. The confederate was carefully rehearsed to respond appropriately in the chair. The subjects were randomly assigned to three conditions. In the model condition, the patients sat behind a one-way viewing screen and observed the confederate-model being treated for six 5-minute sessions over a three-week period. In control condition I, the no-model desensitization condition, subjects sat behind the one-way screen, again for six sessions, observing the dentist demonstrating and naming the equipment used in the experimental condition, no model being present. The subjects in control condition II had no prior exposure to the operatory, professional team, or the model.

The dependent measures were based on two scales, an approach and an avoidance checklist respectively. The approach list had seven items in an ascending order from "walked down hall" to "allowed operative." The avoidance list contained eight items (e.g., crying, restless in chair, won't allow treatment), scored on a four-point scale (absent, mild, moderate, and severe). The dentists conducting the treatment and providing the ratings were unaware of the patient's experimental condition.

The rather complex results of this study clearly supported the efficacy of modeling as a means of reducing dental anxiety. Children exposed to the model exhibited more positive behavior than those in control condition II. However, children in control condition I—the no-model viewing condition, were also less anxious than the no-model no-viewing subjects, thereby indicating the value of systematic desensitization.

Using confederates is a very costly procedure and may be given to bias because it is very difficult to keep the behavior of the confederates constant across all subjects. Wroblewski, Jacob, and Rehm (1977) overcame this problem by using videotapes. This experiment also had three conditions. In what the authors called the "symbolic modeling with relaxation" condition, anxious adult patients were given relaxation training on the first session. During the next five sessions, they were given further relaxation instructions, and then they watched 19 videotaped scenes recorded in a dentist's surgery depicting progressively more anxiety provoking dental situations. Subjects in the "symbolic modeling only" condition were presented with the same videotaped hierarchy, but without the relaxation instructions. The third condition was a control group labeled "attention placebo" in which subjects saw two video tapes, one of a dental student interviewing a patient about his social and medical history, dietary habits, and other matters related to dental health; the second tape showed an empty dental chair.

The results showed that the group exposed to symbolic modeling combined with relaxation improved the most on the behavioral measure of seeking dental care, followed by the modeling-only group. The control group showed the least change.

In another study on the effect of modeling, Melamed, Weinstein, Hawes, and Katin-Borland (1975) assigned 14 children to two groups. The experiment subjects watched a 13-minute videotape of a 4-year-old child coping with anxiety during a dental visit. The child was verbally rewarded for cooperative behavior and given a trinket at the end of the session. Children in the control group did not see the film but were given a drawing task instead. The results indicated that children who saw the modeling videotape were more cooperative and showed significantly less disruptive behavior than children in the control group. There is thus consistent support in the literature for the efficacy of modeling as a method for reducing dental anxiety.

Perceived Control and Anxiety Reduction

It has been suggested that one reason why dental patients are anxious is because they do not have control over what is happening to them. To test this hypothesis, several studies have been conducted in which patients are provided with a signaling device such as a button that activates a red light and a buzzer. The patients are invited to press the button if they wish to communicate with the dentist or if they wish the dentist to pause so that they can rest for a while. A review of this literature by Corah, Bissell, and Illig (1978) and Corah, Gale, and Illig (1979b) reveals conflicting results. In some studies dental patients in "control" of the situation showed less arousal and anxiety than an appropriate comparison group (Wardle, 1983). Other studies have found greater arousal in the "perceived control" condition. And in some studies (e.g., Corah, 1973; Corah, Gale, and Illig, 1979b) no differences were found. The precise role of perceived control in the dental situation has not been identified and further research is needed to explore what intuitively seems like a good idea but so far has eluded unequivocal empiric confirmation.

Biofeedback and Anxiety Reduction

In an interesting development, Carlsson, Linde, and Ohman (1980) have combined desensitization and biofeedback to train phobic patients. The subjects were shown a series of progressively more fear-provoking scenes on a television screen, ranging from a dental nurse seen talking on the telephone to make an appointment, to the dentist using a drill. The patients were given a switch by means of which they could stop and start the tape at will. Subjects were also connected to an EMG feedback device that measures and visually displays muscle tension for biofeedback training. Patients were taught to relax, and then desensitization and biofeedback relaxation training were carried out. Thus, if the EMG feedback device indicated tension, the patient was instructed to stop the tape showing the dental scene that had aroused the anxiety. The training continued until all scenes could be watched without increases in tension. When all the distressing stimuli could be tolerated, dental treatment was discussed with the patients and they were shown actual instruments. During the first appointment, which included an injection of a local anesthetic, patients were allowed to use the tension feedback device if they wished. The results showed that a range of 4 to 11 hourly sessions was needed before dental treatment could commence, with a mean of 7.2 sessions. However, dental treatment was possible with only minor problems for all patients, and all of them recorded a reduction in dental anxiety. Similar results were obtained in a subsequent study (Berggren and Carlsson, 1984), in which 21 out of 24 patients with severe dental fear were successfully treated using this technique. According to the authors, an important element in the therapeutic process is the biofeedback component, which teaches patients how to identify tension, shows them ways of controlling it, and gives patients objective information about their progress. This latter aspect is important because it increases motivation to continue what is quite a distressing experience for phobic patients.

Studies of Oral Hygiene Programs Based on Learning Theory Principles

In addition to reducing dental anxiety and increasing general cooperativeness among dental patients (Stokes and Kennedy, 1980), another major practical aim has been to persuade people to adopt and maintain improved oral hygiene habits. Perhaps the most important of these is having clean teeth, something that in theory can be easily achieved by effective tooth-brushing. However, many people either do not regularly clean their teeth, or do not do so effectively. For instance, Macgregor and Rugg-Gunn (1986) have developed a method for studying toothbrushing in which they ask volunteers to brush their teeth and then film them through a semi-silvered mirror above the washbasin. Such a procedure is superior to direct observation because it provides a permanent record that can then be subsequently studied in a systematic way. Studies of toothbrushing behavior routinely reveal that many people are not very good at it from a dental hygiene point of view, and could benefit from instruction and training to improve their performance.

Although many schools conduct dental health programs based on lectures and demonstrations, these seem to have little effect on the cleanliness of children's teeth. This prompted Swain, Allard, and Holborn (1982) to develop an instruction technique based on behavior modification principles which they called the "Good Toothbrushing Game." Forty-five elementary school children participated in the program, which was run in their school. All the children were examined before the study began to establish their baseline in dental health, including the cleanliness of their teeth. The children were then issued with a dental kit containing a toothbrush, toothpaste, and disclosing tablets, and were also given a lecture and demonstration in oral hygiene.

The children were randomly assigned to two teams and told that they were participating in a daily class game, the object of which was to be the team that had the cleanest teeth. Each day four children from each group were randomly selected to represent their team and have their teeth checked, no one knowing in advance when they would be checked. The winning team had their names posted on the bulletin board, the children were praised for achieving a good score, and they also received feedback about the areas they did not brush well (e.g., "You did not properly clean the inside of your bottom teeth"). The results showed that the childrens' oral hygiene improved markedly while the "Good Toothbrushing Game" was being played, and that this effect persisted when the children were followed up nine months after the program had ended.

In a French study (Kerebel, Le Cabellec, Daculsi, and Kerebel 1985; Kerebel, Le Cabellec, Kerebel, and Daculsi, 1985), 244 children in four schools participated in a program aimed at improving their oral hygiene. What is interesting about this study is that it used a quasi-experimental design. Half of the children were given detailed instructions in toothbrushing, and then brushed their teeth at school every day after lunch. The three-minute toothbrushing was supervised by dental students. In addition to daily supervised toothbrushing, prophylactic treatment was provided every two months, during which the teeth were cleaned and polished. The rest of the children served as a control group, receiving neither oral hygiene instruction nor prophylactic treatment. The study was carried out over three years, and showed that on a variety of measures such as plaque index and prevalence of caries, the oral hygiene of the experimental group was significantly better than that of the control group. The authors conclude that oral hygiene instruction alone, or purely mechanical plaque-control do not have much impact on oral health. What is needed is to motivate children to improve their oral hygiene. The backbone of this study was the daily supervised toothbrushing during school hours, which apparently led to a permanent increase in oral hygiene motivation, and which generalized to the home setting.

Studies such as these confirm what educational psychologists have been saying for a long time, namely that active, behaviorally based learning is much more effective than passive, cognitive, information based instruction, particularly if the aim is to change or instill some form of behavior (e.g., Furnham and Bochner, 1986). Learning by doing not only motivates the student, it also gives instant feedback and hence greatly facilitates the acquisition of a particular skill. Combined with encouragement and reinforcement, active learning by doing is a very effective way of teaching oral hygiene.

Summary and Conclusion

The learning theory conceptualization of dental anxiety has clear implications for the development of methods to reduce dental apprehension. Over the last 15 years there has been an increase in the use of behavior modification techniques in the treatment of dental aversion. Nevertheless, research evaluating the efficacy of these techniques has been sparse, and until recently, largely impressionistic and anecdotal. However, well conducted, relatively sophisticated experiments, using adequate samples of both children and adults, are now beginning to appear in the literature. These studies indicate that the various behavior modification techniques, either singly or in combination, do have a significant impact on dental anxiety, resulting in reduced levels of dental aversion. These findings, however, do not necessarily confirm the learning theory model because the various treatment procedures tend to be confounded with the establishment of a personal relationship between the dentist and the patient. A dentist who relaxes, desensitizes, or shows a model to a patient is also indicating concern for the patient as a person, and a caring attitude for the patient's well-being. It is possible that the crucial variable is the quality of the relationship, and that the actual procedures play a subsidiary role to that relationship.

Traditional learning theory emphasizes the *mechanics* of the treatment (the hierarchies, the muscle relaxation, the imitation of the model) and has little to say about the *interpersonal* context in which these procedures are enacted. The experiment has yet to be done in which the mechanical treatment variables are kept constant, and interpersonal variables such as warmth, trust and respect toward the dentist-behaviorist are systematically varied. Consequently, the theoretic explanation regarding the efficacy of behavior modification techniques in dentistry is incomplete—the methods work, but why they do work is subject to debate. However, the literature does have clear practical implications for the reduction of dental aversion: behavior modification techniques, carried out in the context of a warm, personal relationship between the dentist and the patient, do significantly reduce dental anxiety at the time of the treatment, and for many patients this improvement represents a permanent change in their orientation toward dentistry.

One problem with adopting a behavior modification stance is that it may lead to construing dental anxiety as a phobia in the same way that fear of heights is considered to be a phobia. Taking a phobic view of dental aversion in turn implies that these fears are baseless or irrational. Such a conclusion is not warranted. Certainly, some patients do have a phobia and their fears can legitimately be described as irrational. However, as a study conducted by the author and reported in Chapter 6 has shown, the great majority of patients respond quite rationally to the dental situation. They selectively fear those procedures that hurt or look as if they ought to be painful, they tolerate the less abrasive procedures, and their pain and fear experiences are affected by the extent to which they like and trust their dentists. Thus, to view dental fear primarily as irrational and phobic can lead to quite misleading and erroneous conclusions about the nature and origins of dental aversion, and about the appropriate therapeutic measures to combat it. Although the learning theory model does not necessarily categorize dental aversion as a phobia, many practitioners make that equation. It is not difficult to see why that should be so. Dentists, like most other people, like to be liked, and don't like being disliked (Rubin, 1973). Consequently, there is a tendency for dentists to attribute the negative behavior of their patients to some condition within the patient rather than blaming themselves or their discipline. Both psychoanalysis and learning theory provide this convenient means of avoiding accountability. By labeling the aversive behavior of patients as "irrational," even they escape blame as people cannot be held responsible for their irrational acts. This cozy arrangement takes care of the problem of who is responsible for any unpleasantness—no one—but it lacks scientific substance and obscures the actual dynamics of the dentist-patient relationship. This will be the topic of the next chapter.

6
Social Psychology and Patient Management

This chapter starts out with a brief account of the major theoretic orientations in psychology, leading to a description of the social-psychologic perspective of human behavior. Then, some studies of the dentist-patient relationship grounded in this perspective will be reviewed, followed by the original report of a major Australian study conducted by the author. Throughout, the implications of this literature on patient management are considered.

Models of Human Behavior

Contemporary psychology, being a relatively young discipline, lacks the unity of some of the more established areas of knowledge. Most psychologists would agree that theirs is the science of behavior and experience, but there is a great deal of disagreement about what those terms mean, what aspects of behavior or experience should be emphasized, and what methods should be used in measuring and defining these phenomena. Furthermore, psychology is one of the least neutral of all the sciences because its topic is humankind itself and almost all of psychology's statements and findings have philosophic, value-laden connotations. There is another sense in which the debate is not academic. As we have already seen in previous chapters, how people view human nature directly affects how they conduct themselves in the world of affairs, including the management of a dental practice.

In psychology there exist three major divergencies and countless minor ones. The term "divergency" is being used here in preference to the more conventional "dichotomy" because the differences in perspective represent variations in emphasis rather than mutually exclusive constructions of reality. In a general sense all of the points of view are correct because they all refer to events or constructs that have an empiric base. However, each point of view has its own special domain of utility, both with regard to providing suitable explanations for phenomena as well as suggesting a practical course of action. The problem arises when a particular perspective is applied in an inappropriate domain, or more seriously, when there is an attempt to use the principle to explain all behavior and experience. To date, there is no single explanatory system in psychology analogous say to the law of gravity in physics, or Einstein's extension of this law to MC^2. This lack of general laws of behavior has bothered many psychologists because of their (mistaken) belief that a discipline must have a set of universal principles if it is to attain the status of a science (Koch, 1981). In turn, this has led a number of writers in fruitless pursuit of what Allport (1954) called a "simple and sovereign" theory of human behavior, an unattainable goal given the present state of knowledge.

In evaluating a theory, the correct question to ask is not if it is true, but whether it is useful: What does it explain at what levels of generality, and what effective action does it predict at what levels of specificity? Questions about the existential veridicality of a theory can safely be left to the philosophers, allowing us to accept the simultaneous presence of several theoretic perspectives in psychology and the absence of any one overriding universal framework. Let us now look at the three major divergencies in psychology.

Body or Mind

Probably the longest standing argument has been between the physiologists and the mentalists, a problem inherited from the body-mind issue in philosophy (Scher, 1962). Today no one denies that human beings are biologic as well as psychologic and social animals (Aronson, 1976). There is clear evidence that the biochemic, glandular, central nervous system, brain and other physical functions all interact and play an important role in how we feel, what we do, and what we know (Ohman, 1981). The argument has shifted into the following three issues:

1. *Physiological primacy.* Are physiologic variables the primary causes of psychologic events? The simple answer is, yes sometimes, but not necessarily so. For instance, psychologic events such as anxiety can cause physiologic changes such as the growth of an ulcer (Beecher, 1972). Emotional stress has been implicated in the myofascial pain-dysfunction syndrome (Greene and Laskin, 1974). Biofeedback techniques can alter heart rate, blood pressure, and a host of other responses once thought to be governed by the autonomous nervous system and hence not amenable to conscious control (Basmajian, 1979; Birbaumer, Elbert, Rockstroh, and Lutzenberger, 1981; Yates, 1975). However, it would be just as misleading to adopt a position of

psychologic primacy—the belief that mind always prevails over matter. Many physical and some mental diseases do have a clear physical origin (Hutt and Gibby, 1961). So do some mood states, of which a good example is the depression and confusion some women experience due to hormonal changes associated with the female menopause. The answer therefore is that most behavior is the joint outcome of an interaction between psychologic and physiologic variables, neither of which can be considered as necessarily primary, a view that has been called the holistic approach, where the individual is regarded as "a unit, a whole" (Woodworth, 1959, p. 231).

2. *Reductionism.* In order to *really understand* behavior, is it necessary to reduce it to its physiologic components? This is the doctrine of reductionism, which states that all psychologic phenomena can and should be reduced to their physiologic base (for a brief but highly readable review of this issue see Underwood, 1957, pp. 226–232). Most social psychologists reject reductionism on the grounds that such transformations are inappropriate, impossible given the present state of the art, and probably impossible in principle given the interaction and reciprocal effects of psychologic and physiologic processes. The sorts of topics that social psychologists are interested in highlight the absurdity of strict reductionism. For instance, how would one go about translating morale in the work place, attitude change, racial prejudice, or group conformity to its physiologic "foundations," and what would one gain from such a reduction? There are other topics, though, such as dental anxiety, where it may be quite useful and possibly essential to take into account parallel bodily changes, not because the body is somehow absolutely primary, but because in that particular context bodily changes do play a large role and can be measured with existing procedures and instruments.

The most general refutation of reductionism rests on the principle that there are different domains of discourse, each with its own self-contained "language." Human beings can be studied from many different perspectives. Physiologists study the biochemistry, neurology, the nerves, glands, hormones, genes, and brain cells that constitute the elements in these physical systems. Psychologists study the beliefs, motives, fears, aspirations, and other mental elements that constitute the mind of human beings. Sociologists study how individuals aggregate into groups, and the elements of their discourse are the social classes, trade unions, ethnic communities, and other collectivities of human life. Each domain has its own set of concepts, explanatory principles, and implications for action. It is neither useful nor appropriate to explain phenomena in one domain in terms of the discourse of another domain, and it can be particularly misleading to view the physiologic system as primary. However, when more than one domain of discourse impinges on a problem, as is often the case, then an explanation invoking both domains will be superior to an explanation based on only one set of principles, provided of course that each explanation is offered on its own terms and not as a translation.

3. *Within or between skins.* The third major divergency has been the argument about whether to seek the explanation of behavior inside the person or in the situation. It is a running issue in psychology and we have already encountered it earlier in various parts of this book. The question cuts across all other divergencies including the psychosomatic and reductionism issues, and many regard it as the most important single unresolved problem in psychology today (Endler and Hunt, 1968; Endler and Magnusson, 1976). To recapitulate, one point of view asserts that behavior is primarily determined by "within-skin" characteristics, by the structural aspects that a person can be thought of as possessing. The term "personality" expresses this idea, and refers to the enduring psychologic traits that presumably distinguish and characterize a person in the same way that physical traits such as height, eye color, and body build do. These traits in turn are assumed to have developed as a consequence of the person's genetic make up interacting with the experiences of the individual's life history. We can refer to this approach as "within-skin" because it assumes that a person's behavior is the product of the individual's internal makeup. This view is shared by physiologic psychologists, who tend to emphasize inherited and physically based determinants of psychologic processes; psychoanalysts, who construe all behavior as being the reenactment of the individual's original resolution of the anal, oral, and oedipal conflicts; and behaviorists, who construe acts as stemming from the internalized habits that individuals carry around with them. Incidentally, it is unlikely that these three groups of scholars would agree on any other substantial question relating to behavior, illustrating how the within/between-skin controversy does tend to cut across the major issues in psychology.

The contrasting view states that behavior is governed largely by the situation, particulary the social situation or behavior setting that is the context for the act. This view has been called "between-skin" because an important ingredient in any situation is the presence of other people, who those people are, and what their relationship is to one another. We will return to this issue in the next section.

There is a good deal of experimental evidence in support of the view that situational factors play an important role in the determination of behavior. We have already described the experiments using a simulated prison (Haney, Banks, and Zimbardo, 1973; Lovibond, Mithiran, and Adams, 1979) which showed that subjects given the task of either guard or prisoner very soon began to act appropriately to their assigned roles. Many other studies can be cited that make a similar point. For example, research in the field of littering and vandalism has found that people scatter litter not because of some trait of vandalism but because some situations are more conducive to destruction and littering than others, particularly places that have already been littered or where subjects have seen someone else destroy or litter (Finnie, 1973; Geller, Witmer, and Tuso, 1977; Jorgenson and Dukes, 1976; Krauss, Freedman, and Whitcup, 1978; Zimbardo, 1969).

The Social-Psychologic Perspective

Roles

The principles of group dynamics are the basis for the social-psychologic perspective of human behavior. All groups have or develop a structure so that there tends to be a division of labor whenever people congregate for a purpose. The division of labor has been conceptualized through the notion of a social role. In informal groups, as in formal ones, the respective roles tend to be clearly defined. In traditional households, for example, one person may do the washing up while another dries, one the mowing while the other does the laundry, one the cooking and cleaning while the other the providing. These roles, indeed all roles, are constantly changing as societies change, either gradually or rapidly. The concept of a role, however, remains, even though its contents may change.

Human beings are social animals (Aronson, 1976), living their lives in the company of other people, hermits and shipwrecked mariners excepted. There are a great many groups to which individuals can belong, the most common types of associations being the work, family, recreational, political, educational, and religious bodies. In addition to their function, groups can also be distinguished according to how formal or informal they are, and the steepness of their internal hierarchy.

In formal groups, the division of labor tends to be more explicit than in most informal groups. In any commercial enterprise there will be many functions, reflected in the different divisions of the company. Some will be engaged in manufacture, others in selling, advertising, or coordinating, each person having an allotted specialty in the total mosaic. There is more to it, however, than just carrying out a task. Research has shown that people do not just do a job, they become it in the sense that it enters into their identity. Studies asking people who they are invariably show that individuals identify themselves in part by their occupation—"I am a lawyer, taxi driver, dentist," particularly when they are interacting with a person occupying the counter-role, in the present example client, passenger, patient (Secord and Backman, 1964).

Hierarchy and Status

The division of labor in both formal and informal groups is seldom neutral with respect to status. The most universal distinction is between the role of leader and that of follower (Gibb, 1954). Most groups, including highly informal and peer groups, have someone who functions as a leader or decision maker, even if there is no formal title bestowed on such an individual, or when a supposedly nonhierarchical title such as "coordinator" is used. Formal groups usually openly acknowledge the function of leader, and the people exercising that role have titles such as chairman, captain, manager, producer, and the like.

A hierarchy implies relative status for the individuals participating in that group. Even in the most informal and democratic of groups the persons exercising leadership have greater status than ordinary members. In formal groups the relative status is reflected in differences in privileges, remuneration, badges of rank, and conditions of work (Packard, 1961). In highly structured organizations such as the army, church, or civil service, every person has a precise place in the hierarchy, as do citizens of societies where a caste system prevails.

Norms

A role not only defines a person's place in the group, it also specifies that person's rights and obligations vis-à-vis other persons in the group, or more accurately, other persons occupying particular role positions. A Captain is supposed to salute a Major irrespective of who the senior officer is.

Most roles form part of a role set: husband-wife, father-son, manager-employee, manager-general manager. The same person at different times will be required to enact various roles, in this example that of husband, father, supervisor, and junior, and in each case the required behavior will be quite different.

Society can be thought of as an interlocking matrix of role sets. A particular relationship will work if the persons in that role set agree about their reciprocal rights and obligations. The crucial idea here is the notion of mutual agreement. Some relationships seem very odd to the outside observer. Most of us know of married couples where one person may be seen to be behaving abominably, yet the marriage survives. In extreme cases this could be due to a masochist having married a sadist, with each person obtaining from the liaison precisely what they are looking for. More commonly, the couples would have worked out their own definition of what constitutes an equitable relationship, a subjective assessment at the best of times.

Most interpersonal conflict arises due to the participants disagreeing about what each person can legitimately expect the other to do. For example, an executive may expect his secretary to serve him with tea, whereas the secretary may feel that this is not part of the duties of that office. Social power as distinct from coercive power is normative in the sense that the role contains the obligation to behave in a certain way towards persons in specific counter-roles. A person who takes on a particular job knows that there is an explicit agreement to obey the instructions of the supervisor insofar as they relate to the work role. In the dental surgery, a nurse knows and accepts that she has to carry out the professional duties assigned to her by the dentist; but she may refuse to do the shopping, or go to the dentist's house at the weekend to weed the garden, as that is not part of the role of a nurse.

Industrial disputes are often about changing the reciprocal rights and obligations of the participants. The campaign for shorter hours is a case in point, its purpose being to vary the norms about what is an accepted definition of the working week. Other disputes have the aim of changing the norms relating to what constitutes the legitimate exercise of social power in the work place. For example, in many industrial settings workers are now demanding to be consulted about decisions affecting them, a demand that managers often interpret as a threat to their authority (Bochner, Ivanoff, and Watson, 1974). In role theory terms, the managers and workers no longer agree that it is the legitimate right of a manager to give an order simply because of the role position the manager occupies. There are armed forces in western Europe that now have trade unions for their members, concerned with issues such as defining the legitimate exercise of authority in a modern army.

Some social roles have rather special normative expectations attached to them. For instance, a male medical doctor while in his surgery may ask a female patient to undress, and she will do so without a qualm. If a solicitor made the same request of a female client, or a dentist asked his patients to disrobe, it is unlikely that the request would be complied with. This is an extreme example of social power that is normatively based and role-linked, but most roles have this characteristic to some extent. Dentists are no exception, as we shall now consider.

The Norms of the Dental Surgery

The dental surgery is a special setting with its own role-related rules. The mutual rights and obligations of the dentist and the patient govern the interaction. Presumably all dentists and most patients know what these are. As the dentists are the ones who would have made the rules in the first place, it can be assumed that they would consider the norms appropriate. Less is known or can be assumed about the extent to which patients accept their rights and obligations and the rights and obligations of the dentist, the extent to which they regard the situation as a legitimate exercise of social power. However, role theory suggests that patient acceptance of the dental situation may not be total. The problem is that individuals performing the role of dentist inevitably break two norms widely adhered to outside of the surgery. The first is the norm about not causing pain. In ordinary circumstances most people do not expect to inflict pain on others or have pain inflicted on them. That norm is often broken in the dental relationship. In that sense the dental surgery is an extraordinary setting with unusual rules that many participants may never fully understand or accept, including some dentists. This is probably the real explanation for the many problems encountered in the dental situation, variously labeled as transference by the psychoanalysts and phobic behavior by the learning theorists.

The second norm invariably broken in the dental surgery is the intrusion of the dentist into the personal space of the patient. This is an aspect on which both psychoanalysis and learning theory tend to be silent, yet is a major feature of the dental situation.

Personal Space

Surrounding each person is an invisible bubble that constitutes that individual's personal space (Sommer, 1969). Human beings experience stress if another person intrudes into their portable territory. However, the size of the bubble and the definition of what constitutes an act of invasion depends on who the transgressor is, and the relationship between the "invader" and the "owner" of the territory. As Hall (1966) has found, there are at least four zones of interpersonal distance.

The first is the intimate distance zone, ranging from zero to 18 inches, and is the characteristic spacing for people engaged in lovemaking, comforting, nursing, and other intimate activities. Admission to this zone is reserved for spouses, lovers, and close friends. When strangers are forced into involuntary intimate distance such as in elevators or crowded trains, they find the experience very stressful.

The second zone is the personal distance region, extending from 1½ to 4 feet away from the individual, and is the characteristic spacing for chatting, gossiping, playing cards, and generally interacting with friends and acquaintances. Discomfort is felt if strangers intrude into this space, and also if friends space themselves too far away, outside the limits of the zone.

Next is the social distance zone, 4 to 12 feet in extent, and is the characteristic spacing in formal settings such as the office, in the professional rooms of doctors, lawyers, accountants, and other practitioners, and in shops, television interviews, and wherever people enact their formal roles. Again discomfort occurs if the norm if broken, if the lawyer sits too close to the client or the shop assistant stands too close to the customer.

The last region is the public distance zone, ranging from 12 to 25 feet, and is the characteristic spacing of official, ceremonious occasions such as the formal dinner, church service, courtroom, parliament, political rally, and the university lecture, particularly where there is a large status difference between the speaker and the audience. Embarrassment is often felt when there is an involuntary coming together of such personages with their clients, for example when a student meets a professor in the cafeteria, or a member of the public encounters the distinguished after-dinner speaker in the wash room.

The general principle of spacing is that the "correct" interpersonal distance depends on two things, the nature of the *activity* that the persons are engaged in, and the nature of the *relationship* existing between them. Neither of these conditions are necessarily fixed. For example, strangers on a long train journey thrown together in a crowded compartment may redefine their mutual relationship by introducing themselves to each other. The enforced proximity will then become more appropriate and bearable because it now exists between acquaintances rather than strangers. The accommodation in the dental surgery probably follows a similar principle.

The surgeon for much of the time will be operating within the intimate distance zone, thereby breaking the norm unless the dentist is closely related to the patient. To tolerate this intrusion the patient will have to be able to redefine the relationship. It should follow that a patient who likes, respects, and admires the dentist will find it much easier to suspend the normal reaction to territorial invasion than a hostile, resentful, or suspicious patient.

It will be recalled that the psychoanalysts interpreted patient resistance to dental treatment as reflecting hidden anxieties about oral/vaginal penetration, rape, and homosexual attack. A much more plausible account, supported by a good deal of evidence, suggests that what patients really react to is the invasion of their personal space, in particular the breaking of norms about activities taking place in the intimate interpersonal distance zone. Likewise, the anxiety that dentists sometimes experience can be attributed to their norm breaking by repeatedly intruding into the intimate zones of persons to whom they are not closely attached.

Reinforcements and Relationships

As we saw earlier in this book, the learning theory model asserts that the behavior of human beings is controlled by reinforcement, either through the contiguous association of stimuli (classic conditioning) or by rewarding desired behaviors and punishing undesired acts (instrumental conditioning). There is no doubt that both techniques work. Most animal training is based on the principle of instrumental conditioning. You can teach a dog to sit up by giving it a biscuit each time it performs the desired response, just as you can teach a cat not to scratch the upholstery by belting it each time the claws come out. Indeed, highly elaborate circus routines are built up in the same way. It therefore seems plausible that the behavior of human beings likewise is controlled and modified by reward and punishment. This is a widely held belief and many of the institutions in society are based on its rationale. Most child rearing is founded on this principle. The legal and penal systems depend on it, assuming that fines and jail sentences will deter people from stealing, speeding, going on strike, or killing their spouses. The education system assesses students in the belief that good grades or the fear of bad ones will make everyone study harder. Many other examples could be given of institutions and practices that make the assumption that behavior is controlled by its reinforcing contingencies.

Unfortunately the evidence in real life, as distinct from the laboratory or the armchair, suggests that the principle of reinforcement is somewhat lacking. The jails are full of people who have been there before, the speed limit is largely ignored, juvenile delinquency is rife, and students do not respond to the grading system as expected. Why is this so? The social-psychologic perspective suggests that it is not the rewards and punishments per se that control behavior but *who* is doing the rewarding or punishing. In other words, the quality of the relationship between the source of the reinforcement and its recipient is an important mediating variable. This principle suggests the hypothesis that rewards emanating from a person who is liked, respected, or admired will have quite a different impact than rewards coming from a person who is disliked or distrusted.

There is a good deal of experimental evidence to support this hypothesis. In a series of studies Jones (1964) found that positive acts by a disliked person will be seen by the recipient as attempts at ingratiation. Mann (1974) found that spectators at a football game who supported the losing team, overestimated the number of free kicks awarded to the winning team, were more critical of the umpire, thought the game was dirtier, and rated the standard of the game lower than supporters of the winning team. Winkler and Taylor (1979) telephoned voters just prior to the 1976 American presidental election, asking them who they thought would win and whom they preferred to win. The subjects were then contacted again immediately after the election, and asked why Carter rather than Ford had won. The results showed that Carter supporters attributed the win to Carter's personal characteristics, whereas Ford supporters regarded the outcome as due to chance. Numerous other studies confirm that "facts" are seldom neutral, but practically always interpreted in relation to the source of the statement (who said it) and the preexisting attitude of the listener to the speaker and the issue (Bochner and Insko, 1966).

Thus with the exception of extreme exchanges such as violence, interpersonal acts are seldom intrinsically rewarding or punishing. Rather, the actions take on their reinforcing properties from the source of the act and the quality of the relationship between the actor and the recipient. This principle has an important bearing on the management of dental patients. The implication is that patients who have a personal relationship with their dentist, and who admire, trust, and like their dentist, will put a more positive interpretation on the acts and words of their surgeon than patients whose relationship is poor. In specific, practical terms, patients enjoying a good rapport with their dentist should experience less fear, anxiety, pain, and discomfort; attend more frequently, listen more carefully to the dentist, and follow instructions about dental hygiene; and be less resentful about the financial cost of dental care. Some of these hypotheses will now be examined with reference to the empiric literature. The next section contains a selected review of studies conducted from the perspective of the social psychology of the dental surgery.

Studies of the Social Psychology of Dentistry

Most of the studies of the social psychology of dentistry consist of recommendations about how dentists should behave toward their patients (e.g., Grainger, 1972). However, generally the authors do not provide direct empiric evidence regarding the efficacy of these procedures in improving patient behavior. At best, the prescriptions are based on analogy. For example, Deneen, Heid, and Smith (1973) argue that the same interpersonal qualities known to be effective in counseling and psychotherapy should also facilitate the dentist-patient relationship. The authors identify empathy, respect, genuineness, and warmth as the core conditions transcending and affecting the outcome of any helping relationship including the dental one. However, no direct evidence is presented in favor of what amounts to a very sweeping generalization. Deneen et al. recommend that dentists should become active listeners and attenders. Specifically, they should learn how to make effective eye contact with their patients, respond with appropriate head nodding, maintain a relaxed posture, and indicate by their verbal responses that they are listening to the patient. The authors conclude that a dentist who is perceived as caring will be better able to influence a patient's attitude toward oral health, increase the patient's confidence in the quality of care provided and the patient's respect for the dentist. No data are cited in support of these interesting hypotheses.

Hornsby, Deneen, and Heid (1975) state that in the United States less than 3% of a dental student's professional training is concerned with teaching interpersonal communication skills. These skills are necessary because according to the authors, it is the dentist's responsibility to ensure that patients accept and understand the diagnosis, rationale, and treatment procedures of preventive programs. The authors assume that dentists who have a warm relationship with their patients will be more successful in influencing the behavior and attitudes of their patients. This is a very plausible hypothesis because there is considerable data from a wide variety of studies in social psychology confirming that communicators who are perceived as warm and respected by their audience, are able to change attitudes and influence behavior more readily than persons who are negatively perceived (Hovland, Janis, and Kelley, 1963; Insko, 1967). However, the hypothesis has not been confirmed directly with respect to dentists and their patients in the Hornsby et al. study.

Jackson (1975) provides some specific, practical examples of active listening by the dentist. To establish rapport with the patient the dentist must correctly divine the patient's feelings and then respond appropriately to them. Patients, according to Jackson, will often indicate their feelings in an indirect manner, and the dentist must be sensitive to what the patient is really trying to convey. For example, when a patient says: "I hope this won't take long," the statement probably means "I am nervous about my dental treatment." If this in fact is the case, then it would be insufficient for the dentist to reply merely to the statement (e.g., "No, it will only take a few minutes"). What the patient really wants to hear is reassurance that it won't be painful, cost too much, involve an extraction, or require a local anesthetic. The dentist therefore has to respond to the translation or interpretation of the statement rather than to its overt meaning. The danger of course is that the dentist may misinterpret the hidden meaning (if any) and create unnecessary confusion. However, presumably there are certain regular patterns in the comments that most patients make, whose intent the dentist will come to recognize with experience. Jackson (1975) draws an analogy between the airline pilot constantly monitoring the gauges in the cockpit, and the dentist constantly evaluating the patient's emotional state. For example, the statement "I sure liked Dr. Block. I went to him for 30 years," can probably be translated as "I am not sure that I trust you."

Dentists failing to attend to their patient's feelings can reduce the rapport between them. Take this exchange. Patient: "I see you have a new drill." Dentist: "Yes, a Siemens 242 × 53, a real beauty." According to Jackson, the dentist ignored the real message the patient was sending—anxiety about the drill—and hence did nothing to reduce that anxiety. Or this example. Child: "I hate dentists. I don't want to be here." Dentist: "Come now. Even your little brother didn't mind his check-up. Be a good boy and open your mouth." According to Jackson, this dentist had made a mistake. The child is really saying "I am afraid" and the dentist is passing judgment, in effect saying "Because you are afraid I think you are both childish and bad." Such evaluative statements do not contribute to the establishment of rapport. Nor, according to Jackson, should dentists simply be supportive, such as telling their patients that it is acceptable to feel the way they do but unnecessary. For instance, Jackson disapproves of the following exchange. Patient: "Oh, I wish I did not have to have a new denture, my old one is so comfortable." Dentist: "Many people feel that way at first, but you will get used to it." Jackson suggests that the comment "many people feel that way" and its companion "I often feel the same way myself," are not effective in establishing rapport because the statement takes the focus of attention away from the patient to other people. The present author disagrees. A good deal of research in social psychology (Festinger, 1954; Darley and Latane, 1968) indicates that people are often uncertain about how they should respond to new or ambiguous situations. They take their cue from watching how other people respond. In the dental situation it is not possible to directly observe whether other patients in a similar situation would find the experience painful, irritating, pleasing, acceptable, or unacceptable. In effect, patients are asking themselves and their dentists: "How do other people react to what I am undergoing?" If a dentist can convincingly convey to the patient that other individuals in similar circumstances have found the procedure acceptable, the chances are the patient in question will use that as a guide to what the appropriate response should be.

The type of statement Jackson (1975) approves of most is the understanding statement. Patient: "It is three o'clock already." Dentist: "You are anxious to get away"; or Patient: "Must I have an injection?" Dentist: "You don't like injections." According to Jackson, understanding statements help to establish rapport because they convey to the patient that the dentist really cares about them.

There is no doubt that what has been called a hidden agenda (Hall, 1959,

1966) underlies many conversations taking place in the dental surgery. However, very little empiric research has been conducted to establish the types of exchanges, their relative frequency of occurrence, their latent and overt meanings, and the best way to handle the latent content of patient communications. Jackson's analysis is useful in that it provides the basis for future research. However, his conclusions and suggestions for action regarding patient management should be treated with caution because they are based on impressions, relatively few case studies, and analogy from counseling episodes rather than on solid empiric evidence derived from dental practice. Nevertheless, it is possible to agree with Collett's (1969) conclusion that a permissive, noncritical climate will reduce patients' resistance to saying what they really think. Pendleton and Bochner (1980) found that many patients in general medical practice are inhibited from communicating their anxieties and fears to the physician. In particular there is a great reluctance on the part of medical patients to ask questions about their condition. It is quite likely that similar inhibitions prevent dental patients from discussing their condition with their dentists, in return reducing the opportunity for the dentist to interrogate and instruct the patient. Consequently, anything the dentist can do to create a climate conducive to greater participation by the patient in the proceedings should have a positive effect. The next study is an example of a strategy for turning patients from being passive consumers to becoming active participants in achieving dental health.

Miller (1974) describes a program he has developed to involve patients more in their treatment, a point also made by Weisenberg (1973). The aim is to make patients feel that they are members of the health team. Miller first gets his patients to state their full commitment to a "Preventive Program." Then, patients are given supplies and equipment that is theirs to keep, including items such as: a battery operated slide viewer, photographs that are taken at each visit and given to the patients to enable them to monitor their progress, a working stone model with those tooth surfaces clearly indicating the places that the patient consistently misses when brushing, a torch with a magnifying mirror, a notebook labelled "My Personal Preventive Dentistry Diary," and ample supplies of disclosing tablets, brushes, and floss.

During the program all patients were kept fully informed on the nature and progress of their treatment. In the case of those patients who could not care for their own oral hygiene, the responsibility was delegated to a parent, guardian, relative, nurse, or friend. Unfortunately Miller presents no evidence regarding the efficacy of these procedures in improving dental care and hygiene.

The importance of what dentists say and how they behave, as distinct from the technical procedures they carry out, is convincingly demonstrated in studies evaluating placebo therapy effects (Beecher, 1972). Laskin and Greene (1972) report on a particularly well-conducted investigation using this technique. Fifty patients suffering from myofascial pain dysfunction participated in the study. After the completion of diagnostic testing, they were told that they were suffering from a muscular disorder that was reversible, and reassured of a good prognosis. Then, each patient received a prescription for a placebo drug, accompanied by an enthusiastic endorsement of its potential therapeutic effects. Patients were told that only the university pharmacy had a supply of the drug because it was new, and on payment of a small fee, each subject received a bottle of 30 orange and blue capsules containing sodium lactate. Patients were instructed to take one capsule four times a day for one week, and to report all changes occurring in their condition during that time.

The results showed that 26 of the 50 patients (52%) reported some improvement in their condition after placebo therapy, eight of them to the point where they could be discharged from the clinic. Of the remainder, 20 patients reported no change and 4 claimed that they felt worse. The symptoms that responded most favorably were the subjective ones of pain and tenderness, whereas the more objective problems of clicking and limitation persisted in most of the patients who had these symptoms. A follow-up survey of these patients several years later (Greene and Laskin, 1974) showed that their improved condition had persisted, with most individuals reporting that they were doing quite well. In a later study, Goodman, Greene, and Laskin (1976) administered two mock equilibrations to 25 MPD sufferers and found that 16 (or 64%) of the patients reported a total or nearly total remission of their symptoms.

The general conclusion that can be drawn from these studies is that the psychologic and procedural aspects of the dentist-patient relationship have a strong influence on the outcome of therapy, as well as on the levels of pain and discomfort acknowledged and/or experienced. One specific conclusion casts doubt on Jackson's (1975) contention that supportive statements impede rapport and patient progress. On the contrary, the Laskin and Greene (1972) study provides clear evidence for the efficacy of supportive statements and procedures. It is not suggested that dentists go to the lengths of administering placebo products or treatments to their patients. Indeed, as Beck (1977) points out, there are ethical considerations to be taken into account. Pure placebo therapy involves deception, and its discovery by the patient could lead to a loss of trust and confidence in the practitioner, and a loss of confidence in the profession by the public at large. Another problem relates to the issue of informed consent. In many countries patients now have a legal right to receive complete and understandable information regarding their diagnosis, treatment, and prognosis, so as to be able to either give informed consent or refuse treatment. Pure placebo therapy (which is seldom indicated in dentistry), may be construed to violate both the principle of nondeception and the principle of informed consent. However there is no harm in and a lot to be said for emphasizing the beneficial aspects of the legitimate and routinely carried out procedures in the surgery. For instance, the administration of an anesthetic should be more effective if it is supported by the authoritative statement "In a few minutes you will feel no pain."

Many of the sensations that dental patients experience are ambiguous, in that they can be variously interpreted. Dentists through their words and actions can influence the interpretations that patients make of their internal states and the labels that they attach to these sensations. For example, a patient aware of sharp objects in the mouth can either conclude that a tooth has disintegrated and go into shock, or assume that the chips consist of an old filling, and consider the sensation as a routine aspect of the treatment. The interpretation will almost totally depend on whether the dentist is aware of what is going through the patient's mind ("What is that sensation?"), and on whether the dentist provides the patient with information that leads to a benign rather than a panic stricken interpretation. Schachter and his colleagues (Schachter and Singer, 1962; Schachter and Wheeler, 1962) have conducted several major studies on the labeling of internal states. These experiments confirm that medically lay persons have great difficulty in interpreting their bodily sensations, including toothache (Wozniczka, 1977). In general, people tend to rely on external cues to identify and categorize their feelings. The abominable practice of canned laughter indicates to viewers when they should feel amused. Wise mothers have learned that when their child trips and falls, the best thing to say is: "It doesn't hurt, does it?" Yet this principle is noteworthy by its absence in the descriptions of patient management, despite its rational and empiric appeal. The present author was able to find only one report that used this technique, to reduce negative reactions to dental prophylaxis (the mechanical removal of soft and hard deposits from the tooth surface). In a study with children aged 3 to 12 years, Neiburger (1978) would start the consultation by saying: "Hello, Billy. How are you? Today we are going to clean your teeth with a magic toothbrush and toothpaste." Later in the prophylaxis, the dentist said: "When I brush your teeth it will tickle and make you laugh even more. You don't have to laugh too much, but many children do." The study is poorly designed, and the procedure and results are presented in a confusing manner, but there seems to have been a marked increase in patient cooperation subsequent to the administration of what Neiburger called "suggestion" but what was really a labeling manipulation.

Schachter's ideas, first published in the early 1960s, have been very influential in stimulating research and theorizing in the psychology of emotion, a subject of obvious relevance to an understanding of dental anxiety. A brief description of the current version of the model is therefore in order. Excellent reviews of this literature can be found in Eiser (1986) and Reisenzein (1983).

According to Schachter, an emotion results from the interaction between two processes: physiologic arousal and a thought or cognition about the arousing situation. Physiologic arousal is conceptualized as being emotionally neutral, its main function being to determine the intensity of an emotional state, but not its quality. It is the cognition that determines which emotion, if any, will be experienced. But the mere temporal coincidence of these two components is not sufficient for an emotional state to occur, although arousal and cognition are considered to be the necessary conditions for an emotion to be experienced. To illustrate, if a snake were to suddenly appear in a person's visual field, this perception would arouse the individual but not necessarily produce fear. Fear will only be experienced if the cognition (I see a snake) and the arousal (I feel aroused) are connected and labeled as indicating danger (The snake will bite me and I will die).

More recently, the labeling of arousal has been interpreted in terms of another prominent construct in psychology, the concept of causal attribution (Jones and Nisbett, 1971). To illustrate, an individual will experience an emotion if 1) the person has an appropriate cognition (I see a snake), 2) is aroused by the perception (I feel aroused), 3) makes a causal connection between the two (My arousal is due to having seen the snake), and 4) labels the situation as dangerous (The snake may bite me, and because it could be poisonous I might die). Thus, an emotion is the result of arousal and three cognitions: a perception of a particular object, a causal belief that the arousal was due to the perception of that object, and a belief that the situation is potentially dangerous, or exciting, or erotic, or whatever interpretion is placed on it.

Schachter distinguishes between two ways in which emotions are generated. In everyday, "normal" emotional states, the cues arousing the person also generally provide the cognitive labels for the arousal (I see a snake, I am aroused, I am aware of being aroused, my arousal is caused by the perception of that snake, snakes are dangerous, I am afraid). It is assumed that these cognitive processes occur rapidly and are below the level of consciousness, so that the individual is aware only of the resultant emotional state, in this example fear. A less common and less typical way in which emotional states can arise is when there is a perception of some "unexplained" arousal, an awareness of physiologic arousal for which no immediate causal explanation comes to mind. Examples include physiologic disorders, the consumption of drugs with unanticipated side effects, sleep deprivation, and in the case of dental patients, nonspecific sensations of oral discomfort. When such unexplained arousal occurs, Schachter says that the individual will engage in a causal search process to find a reason for the arousal. This search for a cause is deliberate and conscious, and not automatic as in the case of everyday emotional states, and it ceases as soon as a plausible cause for the arousal has been found. If an emotional source is identified as the cause for the arousal, then the person will experience the corresponding emotion. To illustrate, an unexplained sound in the house will arouse a person. If the person then attributes the arousal to the refrigerator turning itself on, no emotion will result. If, however, the person attributes the arousal to a burglar making an entrance through a window, the individual will experience fear. It is the generation of emotion based on making attributions about nonspecific physiologic arousal that has direct implications for an understanding of some kinds of dental fears.

In summary, the core idea of the model is that what produces emotions is the subjective representation of a situation or an event such as defining it as "dangerous," or "exciting," or "funny"; more generally, that there is an ongoing cognitive appraisal and analysis of the environment fueled by physiologic arousal that leads to various emotional states. Emotion, according to Schachter, is a postcognitive phenomenon. Another basic idea is that physiologic arousal is regarded as being undifferentiated, emotionally nonspecific, so that arousal per se is conceived of as being affectively neutral and only becomes emotionally tinged after being labeled as such. In addition, Schachter distinguishes between physiologic arousal and perceived arousal, the latter rather than the former being regarded as the proximate determinant of an emotion.

One final concept must be introduced, which will bring the discussion back full circle to where it started, namely in the dental surgery. "Unexplained" arousal, that is, arousal for which no obvious cause is apparent, lends itself to being explained in a variety of different ways. When the true source of the arousal is not or cannot be identified, or when the arousal is attributed to a condition that did not or could not have produced it, *misattribution* is said to have occurred. As was mentioned earlier, dental patients may misattribute the cause of their nonspecific sensations to antecedent conditions that elicit fear and anxiety. From the dentist's point of view, the process of misattribution can be used to induce patients to make attributions about their sensations that will lead to positive rather than negative emotions.

Schachter's theory of emotion has generated a great deal of research. For instance, in his review, Reisenzein (1983) cites around 220 empiric studies, and this literature has undoubtedly grown in the meantime. Although, as is the case in most fields, there is controversy about some of the details of the model, there is nevertheless considerable agreement about the main features, particularly in regard to the salient role of the cognitive component in generating emotions. There is no doubt that the theory can account for some of the varieties of dental anxiety, and can be used to generate procedures aimed at reducing such anxiety.

Another way of regarding the labeling and placebo effects is to think of them as instances of the more general process of expectation. Several studies have been done that explicitly look at the effect of expectations on dental fear and anxiety. Kent (1984) administered a Dental Anxiety Scale to 76 dental patients as they arrived for their appointment. He also asked them how much pain they expected to feel on the present visit, and how much pain they expected to feel on future visits. The results showed that high-anxious subjects expected more pain than low-anxious patients. Wardle (1984) approached 51 patients who were waiting to have a tooth extracted, asked them to rate their present level of anxiety, and to indicate how much pain they expected to feel during the injection of the local anesthetic and during the actual extraction. After they had their tooth removed, they were asked again to rate the pain they had experienced during these two procedures. The results showed that fearful patients expected their treatment to be

more painful than fearless patients. However, there was no relationship between the amount of actual pain experienced and anxiety. In other words,
fearless patients were more accurate in predicting levels of pain than fearful
ones. Thus, even if a particular dental experience is likely to be much less
painful than patients anticipate, this may not necessarily influence their expectations the next time round. This may explain why some people, particularly those who are anxious, continue to regard dental treatment as a painful
experience despite modern developments that have greatly reduced the
amount of pain involved. The problem is that even if experience contradicts
expectations, as long as expectations of harm persist so will the anxiety about
the procedures. One implication of this model for the management of dental
anxiety is to change the expectations by providing patients with information
during treatment that the probability of pain will be low. If one can reduce
their expectations of discomfort, chances are this will also reduce their level
of anxiety, thereby setting up a positive spiral that should lead to more veridical cognitions about dental procedures.

At a more general level still, the preceding section refers to the interaction
between cognitive and emotional processes, in particular about thoughts of
varying kinds and anxiety. Some work has been done specifically on the link
between negative cognitions and dental anxiety. Kent and Gibbons (1987)
gave 198 undergraduates a list of eight negative thoughts that sometimes
occur to dental patients, such as "I have thought that any treatment I need
will be very painful," or "When a dentist is drilling a tooth, I have thought
that he will hit a nerve at any moment." Subjects had to indicate by a "yes"
or a "no" whether they ever had any of these thoughts. The subjects also
completed a Dental Anxiety Scale. The results showed that the higher the
subjects' level of anxiety, the more negative thoughts they had. For practical
purposes, whether the thoughts cause the anxiety or vice versa is largely
irrelevant, since this is another instance of a mutually reverberating system
with each element acting on the other in a continuous cycle. Likewise, a
reduction in one aspect should bring about a lessening in the other. Thus, if
the aim is to intervene in the cycle, whether the point of entry occurs in the
cognitive or emotional domains also becomes largely irrelevant, and will depend on the preferences of the therapist and on what is deemed as being more
practicable.

The Kent and Gibbons study drew its rationale from Bandura's (1983)
theory of self-efficacy. It is appropriate to briefly review this theory, as it has
implications for the understanding and management of dental anxiety.

As was discussed elsewhere in this book, anxiety is generally regarded as
having three components, or to be more precise, anxiety is measured by
observing changes in three different domains: 1) the physiologic domain,
where changes in processes such as heart rate, respiratory rate, or sweating
are deemed to be indicative of anxiety; 2) the behavioral domain, where
responses such as restlessness, facial expressions, or avoidance behaviors are
supposed to indicate anxiety; and 3) the cognitive/emotional domain, in

which people are asked whether they feel anxious. Two further assumptions are generally made about anxiety: first, it is assumed that a high correlation exists between the three indices, so that measured levels of anxiety at one level are taken to be indicative of levels of anxiety in the other two domains. As we saw, this assumption is not always supported by the empiric evidence, there being studies showing that physiologic indices do not always correlate with verbal self-reports of anxiety, at least when it comes to dental anxiety (Keys, 1978). The second assumption is that changes in one domain (e.g., the cognitive) will lead to changes in the other two (e.g., the physiologic and behavioral domains). Bandura's theory of self-efficacy is particularly concerned with this second assumption.

Bandura and colleagues (Bandura, 1983; Bandura, Reese, and Adams, 1982) state that peoples' perceptions of their efficacy affect what they choose to do and their likelihood of success. In other words, the beliefs that people have about their ability to perform an act will affect how they regard that act, and what its expected consequences for them might be. For example, drivers who distrust their skill will conjure up outcomes of wreckage and bodily injury, while those confident of their driving abilities will anticipate sweeping vistas and a pleasant relaxing ride. The former driver will fear driving, the latter not. Thus, according to this theory, what makes potentially aversive events fearsome is a perceived inefficacy to cope with them. This has been confirmed in studies showing that people who are led to believe that they can exercise some control over painful stimuli display less anxiety and impairment than those who lack personal control, even though both groups were subjected to the same painful stimulation. People who judge themselves to be inefficacious in managing potential threats, approach such situations with greater anxiety than those who reckon they can cope.

Bandura reports that peoples' internal dialogues—what they are thinking and saying to themselves—mirrors their self-percepts of efficacy or inefficacy. Fearful people believe that their inept coping behaviors will cause disaster. Here are some extracts from a snake phobic thinking aloud while asked to handle a snake: "I may squeeze the snake's head too hard and provoke it to strike me; it can take you by surprise with those slithering unpredictable movements; I'd lose control and drop it." Bandura concludes that fears and expectations of calamity are to a large extent determined by the belief that people will not be able to cope with the situation, that is, with perceived coping efficacy rather than by aspects of the feared object; and that anticipatory fear and phobic thinking can be reduced by training people to cope with the stressful situation, and even more to the point, give them the confidence to believe that they will be able to cope.

This model has clear implications for the reduction of dental anxiety. Catastrophic thinkers, patients who believe that they will be unable to control their thoughts and emotions in a dental situation, are likely to show more anticipatory anxiety, not necessarily because they are more afraid of dental procedures, but because they are more afraid of losing control over their cognitions. According to the theory, then, control over the thoughts may be more important than their contents. This account of dental anxiety may sound a little farfetched, but Bandura cites an impressive amount of evidence for a variety of phobias, supporting this explanation. The practical implication for the management of fearful dental patients is to try and change their cognitions, particularly their self-perceptions about how well they will be able to handle dental stress. This can be done by modifying the internal dialogue that all persons engage in when facing some challenge of problem: "Yes, I can cope with this situation. Yes, I have some self-efficacy to perform this behavior. Yes, I am confident I am going to be able to control myself when I get close to the fearful object." This procedure therefore provides a cognitive adjunct to the more traditional behaviorally oriented methods of relaxation and systematic desensitization commonly used in the treatment of fear (see Chapter 5). But, as we said earlier, the cognitive, emotional, physiologic and behavioral elements all form a complex, interacting system. Provided a positive spiral is set up somewhere in that system, the predicted end results ought to be similar.

Recently, research has begun to appear that takes seriously the notion that the dentist and the patient form a mutually influencing, interdependent, reverberating social system, with each person affecting and being affected by the behavior (or perceived behavior) of the other. Most social interactions have this quality but the mutuality of influence is intensified in relationships that are emotionally charged and physically or psychologically isolated from the outside world. Dental appointments seem to fulfil these conditions rather well. Using this model, Weinstein, Getz, Ratener, and Domoto (1982a; 1982b) have found that the behavior of child patients is systematically related to the management style of the dentist. Twenty-five dentists and 50 children participated in the study, in which all sessions were videotaped. Child behaviors were classified into fearful and nonfearful responses, and related to specific dentist acts. The fearful behaviors included crying, screaming, whimpering, protest, hurt, and discomfort. Four dentist behavior categories were identified: guidance, empathy, physical contact, and verbalization. The results show that providing immediate direction and specific reinforcement tended to be followed by a reduction in the child's fear, as was patting and stroking. Explanations, although frequently used, did not appear to reduce fear. Reassurance was also not effective, although questioning for feelings was. Coercion, coaxing, and put-downs increased fear, as did stopping the treatment to manage the child.

The authors then looked at the other side of the coin to see if patient behavior had any systematic effects on the responses of the dentist. The results showed that dentists tend to respond to a child's fearful behavior with acts that are counterproductive, that is, with rules, coercion, coaxing, reassurance, and put-downs. Nonfearful patient behavior tended to elicit direction and reinforcement from the dentists.

These studies constitute a pioneering attempt to document the existence of and quantify the reciprocal effect of the dentist-patient relationship. Even if some of the details may need modification in the light of subsequent research, these studies have empirically established the principle of interdependence and mutual accommodation between dentist and patient, confirm that a major ingredient in successful patient management is the style adopted by the dentist, and provide clear suggestions consistent with social-psychologic theory as to which style is effective in eliciting cooperative behavior in dental patients.

A Major Australian Study

The present author carried out a large-scale study of the dentist-patient relationship. The study was conducted in Sydney, Australia, and was supported by funds from the Dental Health Education and Research Foundation of the University of Sydney. The experiment will be described in detail, as it has not been previously published.

The aim of the study was to provide empiric support for some of the claims made in the literature. As the review in the preceding pages has shown, there is a widely held belief that the manner in which a patient responds to dental treatment will depend in part on how the patient regards the dentist, which in turn will be affected by how the dentist interacts with the patient and on the quality of the relationship existing between them. However, the literature has at least two major weaknesses: the variables are usually not precisely defined, and the conclusions drawn are often based on folklore rather than empirical evidence. The experiment about to be described has precisely defined independent (antecedent) and dependent (outcome) variables, clearly stated hypotheses derived from theory, a large sample, appropriate controls, and the results were submitted to sophisticated statistical analyses permitting the drawing of unequivocal conclusions.

Introduction and Overview

The method consisted of a structured interview. The interviews were conducted in the waiting rooms of dental surgeries. The subjects were dental patients attending the surgery as part of a regular appointment. All interviews were conducted immediately before the subjects received dental treatment.

Three conditions were systematically varied in the study: a) the type of dental practice, which was either preventive or restorative; b) the socioeconomic status (SES) of the patients, as indicated by the location of the practice in either a high- or a low-income suburb; and c) the gender of the patients.

Four outcome or dependent variables were systematically measured: a) the degree of anxiety aroused by various aspects of dental treatment; b) patients' confidence in their dentists; c) the stereotypes that patients hold about their dentists; and d) patients' factual knowledge about dental hygiene.

The analysis addressed two problems. The first was to determine the anatomy of dental anxiety. What aspects of the dental situation arouse anxiety and to what extent, and do different aspects arouse differing degrees and kinds of anxiety? The second problem was to determine the effect of the three independent variables (type-of-practice, SES, and gender), either singly or in combination, on each of the dependent variables (anxiety, confidence, stereotypes, and knowledge). In addition the effect of age on the dependent variables was also assessed. For obvious reasons, age could not be systematically varied, and was therefore treated as a covariate.

The design of the study is explicitly related to the major hypothesis under examination: that how a patient responds to the stress of the dental situation, and what the patient feels and thinks about the dentist, depends systematically on who the patient and the dentist are—on the patient's gender, age, income, education, etc.; *and* on the characteristics of the dentist, including whether the dentist practices predominantly restorative or predominantly preventive dentistry, the extent to which dental education is provided, the location of the practice, etc. The results confirmed this model of the dental situation, although some of the antecedent variables were found to be more influential than others.

If it is true that the responses of dental patients are a systematic function of the social psychology of the treatment situation, this casts doubt on the widely held belief that patients have a general and irrational fear of dental practice. As we saw earlier, implicit in both psychoanalytic and classic learning theory is the assumption that the dental surgery generates pervasive and undifferentiated anxiety, so that all aspects of treatment, even totally innocuous ones such as the chair or the surgeon's white smock can evoke distress. In contrast, the social-psychologic model expects the dental patient to be far more rational and pragmatic. In particular, the model assumes that patients can distinguish those aspects of the treatment situation that cause pain or are directly associated with pain, from those aspects that cause discomfort but are not painful in the usual sense of that term. The results of the present study conclusively confirmed this hypothesis and have important implications for the management of dental stress, both as experienced by the patient and also by the dentist.

Finally, in contrast to much of the literature in this area, the design of the present study enables conclusions to be drawn that are unequivocal and generalizable. Five limitations characterize the bulk of the literature: a) small samples, affecting the generalizability of the results; b) unrepresentative samples, affecting the generalizability of the results; c) the confounding of subject variables (age, gender, SES, etc.) with type of dentistry, affecting the interpretation of the results; d) an inadequate conceptualization and operationalization of the dependent variable, leading to misleading interpretations;

and e) either an atheoretic survey approach, or a highly constraining theoretic framework such as the psychoanalytic model or a model assuming the existence of learned phobias. The problem with survey-type studies is that they produce a mass of unrelated data that are difficult to interpret. The problem with studies that are too narrowly conceived is that their method usually does not allow the hypothesis to be falsified.

In the present study, the size of the sample was precisely calculated to permit the results to be generalized. The subjects were selected so as to represent the main categories of patients, and the dentists were selected so as to represent the main categories of practitioners. The principal subject and practitioner variables were systematically varied to avoid confounding. The dependent variables were explicitly selected with a view to testing hypotheses about their relationship to the independent variables. Finally, the hypotheses were systematically derived from a general theory of social behavior, and tested with a design that permitted these hypotheses to be either confirmed or disconfirmed in the light of empiric evidence.

Design

The design of the study appears in Table 6.1. Three conditions were systematically varied: a) type of dental practice (preventive or restorative), b) socioeconomic status (SES) of the patients (high or low), and c) gender of patients.

Eight surgeries participated in the study, two in each of the respective type-of-practice by SES conditions. Surgeries were classified as either preventive or restorative from information provided by members of the Dental Health Foundation Research Committee, from information provided by the respective dentists themselves in response to a direct inquiry about the type of practice they conducted, and from observations made by the interviewers. The distinguishing criterion was whether both adults and children were given cleaning instructions and demonstrations, general dental education, and cleaning and fluoridation during each treatment program.

Table 6.1. Design of the Study*

Type of practice	Inter-viewer	Socioeconomic status of suburb[†]			
		High		Low	
Preventive		Dr. PH_1[2.98]	Dr. PH_2[2.48]	Dr. PL_1[5.38]	Dr. PL_2[4.85]
	Ms. N	18 Ms 18 Fs	18 Ms 18 Fs	18 Ms 18 Fs	18 Ms 18 Fs
	Ms. B	18 Ms 18 Fs	18 Ms 18 Fs	18 Ms 18 Fs	18 Ms 18 Fs
Restorative		Dr. RH_1[3.08]	Dr. RH_2[2.48]	Dr. RL_1[5.38]	Dr. RL_2[5.89]
	Ms. N	18 Ms 18 Fs	18 Ms 18 Fs	18 Ms 18 Fs	18 Ms 18 Fs
	Ms. B	18 Ms 18 Fs	18 Ms 18 Fs	18 Ms 18 Fs	18 Ms 18 Fs

*N = 576
†The numbers in brackets indicate the status ranking of the suburbs.

The SES rating of the suburbs in which the respective practices are located was determined according to a scale developed by the Sydney sociologist Congalton (1969). The range of the scale is 1 to 7, the lower the score the higher the standing of the suburb, and vice versa. The actual status score of each suburb appears in Table 6.1 in brackets after each dentist's identifying symbol.

As Table 6.1 indicates, 576 subjects served in the study. The design is completely counterbalanced: half the *Ss* were tested in a preventive, and half were tested in a restorative surgery; half the *Ss* were tested in a surgery located in a high-status suburb, and half in a surgery in a low-status suburb; and the number of males and females was equal in each cell.

Overcoming Surgery-Specific and Interviewer-Specific Effects

Two surgeries were employed in each type-of-practice by SES condition. The reason for the duplication was that if only one surgery per condition had been used, the possibility could not be ruled out that the results were due to attributes specific to that particular surgery, rather than to general factors determined by the respective surgery's type and SES clientele. However, if the results in each cell are based on more than one surgery and no significant differences occur between the surgeries in each condition, then there is a much greater likelihood that the findings reflect general rather than surgery-specific effects.

Two interviewers were employed, each investigator interviewing half of the subjects in each condition. The reason for the duplication was that if only one interviewer had collected all the data, the possibility could not be ruled out that the pattern in the data was affected and hence distorted by the specific attributes of the investigator. However, with two investigators working in parallel, such an explanation becomes less tenable, particularly if an analysis reveals no interexperimenter differences.

Procedure

Subjects were interviewed in the waiting rooms of the surgeries while waiting for their consultation. The dentist and his staff had been briefed on the purpose and method of the study, and they provided full and active cooperation. The interviewer (a young woman) would approach a patient and introduce herself as follows: "My name is (E.N. or M.B.). I am from the Dental Health Research Foundation. We are doing research on attitudes to dental matters. Would you like to take part? It will only take a few minutes, and the results will be completely confidential—your name will not be recorded, and the dentist will not see your responses." Altogether 32 individuals who were approached refused to take part in the study; Ms. N had 17 and Ms. B had 15 refusals.

All patients present in a particular surgery on the day in question were included in the study, provided they satisfied the following criteria: they were between the ages of 20 and 60, had attended that particular surgery at least once in the past, and could speak and write English. Testing continued until the quota of 18 males and 18 females per interviewer per surgery was reached.

The method was a structured interview. *Ss* indicated their answers by marking a questionnaire, or by ticking an alternative on a card that *E* presented to them. All *Ss* were tested individually. Privacy was achieved by *E* and *S* withdrawing to a quiet corner of the waiting room.

Details of the various questionnaires will be described in conjunction with the presentation of the results.

Results and Discussion

Checks on the Manipulations

The SES Manipulation

Subjects were asked to indicate their or their spouses' income on a five-point wage-range scale. The mean income range of the patients in the high SES condition was 3.33, whereas the mean income range of low SES patients was 2.32. These differences are highly significant (t = 16.9; df = 416; p < .001) and provide corroboration for the respective SES of the patients in the two conditions.

The Type-of-Practice Manipulation

Subjects were asked the reason for their attendance at the surgery by means of a card on which they checked whether they were about to receive preventive, restorative, or emergency treatment. After the consultation, the dentist was independently asked what kind of treatment he had just administered, using the same categories. A frequency table of the respective responses by type-of-practice was prepared, and is presented in Tables 6.2 and 6.3. The analysis supports the type-of-practice manipulation because both tables indicate that a significantly higher proportion of preventive dentistry was being carried out in the preventive than in the restorative surgeries.

Checks on Surgery-Specific and Interviewer-Specific Effects

An extensive analysis revealed no significant differences between the parallel surgeries in each cell, on each of the dependent variables. Similarly, no significant differences between the two interviewers were found. These data diminish the possibility that the substantive findings of the study are limited to the particular surgeries sampled and interviewers employed.

Table 6.2. Frequency Distribution of Patients Giving Various Reasons for Treatment in the Two Type-of-Practice Conditions

	Type of practice			
	Preventive		Restorative	
Patient's reasons	N of Ss	%	N of Ss	%
Preventive	110	38	85	30
Restorative	117	41	153	53
Emergency	39	13	32	11
Preventive and restorative	20	7	13	4
Restorative and emergency	2	1	5	2
Total	288	100	288	100

$\chi^2 = 10.31$; df = 4; p < .05.

Table 6.3. Frequency Distribution of Various Types of Treatment Received by Patients in the Two Type-of-Practice Conditions

	Type of practice			
	Preventive		Restorative	
Type of treatment	N of Ss	%	N of Ss	%
Preventive	112	39	65	23
Restorative	129	46	183	65
Emergency	26	9	26	9
Preventive and restorative	13	5	8	3
Restorative and emergency	3	1	1	–
Total*	283	100	283	100

$\chi^2 = 24.02$; df = 4; p < .05.

* Information on 5 Ss in each condition was not available.

Substantive Results

Anxiety in the Dental Situation

Patients' reactions to the dental situation were measured by means of a 25-item "Attitudes to Dental Treatment" scale. The scale consists of 25 statements about dental treatment (e.g., "needles and injections," "when the dentist puts his hand in my mouth"), followed by the phrase "makes me feel" or "I feel." Subjects responded by checking a five-point scale where *1* was labeled "not at all anxious," and *5* was labeled "extremely anxious." The full questionnaire is reproduced on pages 117–118.

Three sets of analyses were performed on the data. The first analysis was concerned with determining the absolute amount of anxiety produced by various aspects of the treatment situation, or in operational terms, the average amount of anxiety for each item on the scale. A second analysis sought

ATTITUDES TO DENTAL TREATMENT

The following items refer to different aspects of dental treatment. Please mark on the corresponding scale the degree to which each of the items make you feel worried, tense, nervous, or anxious.

For example: If the white coat that your dentist wears makes you feel slightly anxious then you would place a mark as follows:

The white coat that my dentist wears makes me feel:

Not at all anxious : 1 : ② : 3 : 4 : 5 : Extremely anxious

1. Bright lights make me feel:
   Not at all anxious : 1 : 2 : 3 : 4 : 5 : Extremely anxious
2. Not being able to see what the dentist is doing makes me feel:
   Not at all anxious : 1 : 2 : 3 : 4 : 5 : Extremely anxious
3. The smell of the surgery makes me feel:
   Not at all anxious : 1 : 2 : 3 : 4 : 5 : Extremely anxious
4. Needles and injections make me feel:
   Not at all anxious : 1 : 2 : 3 : 4 : 5 : Extremely anxious
5. Reclining back in the dentist's chair makes me feel:
   Not at all anxious : 1 : 2 : 3 : 4 : 5 : Extremely anxious
6. The air or suction pump in my mouth makes me feel:
   Not at all anxious : 1 : 2 : 3 : 4 : 5 : Extremely anxious
7. Having the dentist breathing on me makes me feel:
   Not at all anxious : 1 : 2 : 3 : 4 : 5 : Extremely anxious
8. Feeling little bits of teeth and fillings in my mouth makes me feel:
   Not at all anxious : 1 : 2 : 3 : 4 : 5 : Extremely anxious
9. Being unable to move or talk during treatment makes me feel:
   Not at all anxious : 1 : 2 : 3 : 4 : 5 : Extremely anxious
10. When the dentist drills on my tooth I feel:
    Not at all anxious : 1 : 2 : 3 : 4 : 5 : Extremely anxious
11. Having water run in my mouth makes me feel:
    Not at all anxious : 1 : 2 : 3 : 4 : 5 : Extremely anxious
12. Having to keep my mouth open makes me feel:
    Not at all anxious : 1 : 2 : 3 : 4 : 5 : Extremely anxious
13. When the dentist picks at my tooth with a sharp instrument I feel:
    Not at all anxious : 1 : 2 : 3 : 4 : 5 : Extremely anxious
14. When the dentist puts his hand in my mouth I feel:
    Not at all anxious : 1 : 2 : 3 : 4 : 5 : Extremely anxious
15. When the dentist squirts air into my mouth I feel:
    Not at all anxious : 1 : 2 : 3 : 4 : 5 : Extremely anxious
16. When my face and mouth go numb I feel:
    Not at all anxious : 1 : 2 : 3 : 4 : 5 : Extremely anxious
17. Being unable to stop the dentist when it hurts too much makes me feel:
    Not at all anxious : 1 : 2 : 3 : 4 : 5 : Extremely anxious
18. When the room is too hot or too cold I feel:
    Not at all anxious : 1 : 2 : 3 : 4 : 5 : Extremely anxious

19. When the dentist places all his instruments in front of me I feel:
    Not at all anxious : 1 : 2 : 3 : 4 : 5 : Extremely anxious
20. Not being able to swallow comfortably makes me feel:
    Not at all anxious : 1 : 2 : 3 : 4 : 5 : Extremely anxious
21. Having cotton wool in my mouth makes me feel:
    Not at all anxious : 1 : 2 : 3 : 4 : 5 : Extremely anxious
22. Having to keep still makes me feel:
    Not at all anxious : 1 : 2 : 3 : 4 : 5 : Extremely anxious
23. Having the dentist lean over me makes me feel:
    Not at all anxious : 1 : 2 : 3 : 4 : 5 : Extremely anxious
24. Having to have a tooth pulled makes me feel:
    Not at all anxious : 1 : 2 : 3 : 4 : 5 : Extremely anxious
25. The sound of the drill makes me feel:
    Not at all anxious : 1 : 2 : 3 : 4 : 5 : Extremely anxious
26. Are there any other aspects of dental treatment that make you feel anxious, nervous, worried or tense?

to reveal whether the various aspects of the treatment situation clustered together into natural categories. In operational terms, the data were submitted to a factor analysis to determine any groupings among the 25 items. In the third analysis, the responses of individuals in the various experimental conditions were compared to determine the effect of these conditions (e.g., SES or type-of-practice) on anxiety. In operational terms, the 25 scores of each individual subject were reduced to two scores, corresponding with that individual's score on each of the two clusters or factors revealed by the second analysis, and these factor-scores were then used in comparing individuals across the various experimental groups.

What Makes Patients Anxious?

The scores for each statement were summed across all 576 subjects, and an average computed. These data appear in Table 6.4. The statements have been abbreviated and arranged in descending order of anxiety. It is sometimes the case in attitude measurement that subjects are reluctant to use the extreme ends of the scale (Guilford, 1967; Crano and Brewer, 1973; Selltiz, Jahoda, Deutsch, and Cook, 1963). It is therefore reasonable to suppose that a score greater than *3* indicates high anxiety; a score between *2* and *3* indicates moderate anxiety; and a score less than *2* indicates slight anxiety.

Before interpreting these results, it should be noted that the data in Table 6.4 are average results based on the responses of all the subjects irrespective of their SES, gender, age, or type-of-practice. Individual and group differences can be expected to exist, as indeed is indicated by the fairly large standard deviations on some of the items (the standard deviation is a measure of

Table 6.4. Mean Anxiety Scores and Standard Deviations of Items in the "Attitudes to Dental Treatment" Scale

Statements*	Mean	Standard deviation
24. Tooth pulled	3.73	2.36
17. Unable to stop dentist when it hurts	3.37	1.38
10. Dentist drills on tooth	3.28	1.31
25. Sound of drill	3.06	1.42
4. Needles and injections	3.06	1.38
20. Not being able to swallow	2.78	1.25
13. Dentist picks at tooth	2.78	1.26
18. Room too hot or cold	2.04	1.79
12. Keep mouth open	1.96	1.12
8. Bits of teeth and fillings in mouth	1.95	1.14
6. Air or suction pump in mouth	1.95	1.17
16. Face and mouth numb	1.92	1.21
9. Unable to move or talk	1.92	1.10
3. Smell of surgery	1.89	1.16
21. Cotton wool in mouth	1.88	1.10
19. Instruments in sight	1.85	1.18
15. Air squirts in mouth	1.77	1.01
2. Unable to see what dentist doing	1.73	1.00
5. Reclining in chair	1.67	1.02
11. Water run in mouth	1.66	1.00
22. Having to keep still	1.61	1.01
1. Bright lights	1.61	0.90
14. Dentist's hand in mouth	1.60	0.93
7. Dentist breathing on patient	1.47	0.85
23. Dentist leans over patient	1.35	0.79

*The numbers refer to the item's original position in the "Attitudes to Dental Treatment" Questionnaire.

dispersion; the larger the index, the greater the range of differences around the mean score). Thus these data provide a gross picture only, to be refined by subsequent analyses that break these results up into their component parts.

With this proviso, it is clear that not all aspects of the dental situation are threatening, and those aspects that do arouse anxiety are not equally threatening but vary in their impact. As the data in Table 6.4 show, having a tooth pulled, being unable to stop the dentist when it hurts, having a tooth drilled, and needles and injections create a good deal of anxiety, whereas the dentist leaning and breathing over the patient, putting his hand in the patient's mouth, and the bright lights in the surgery are not particularly anxiety arousing. In the middle of the spectrum are the instruments and other sources of discomfort such as the suction process, the feeling of numbness, and the inability to move or talk. What emerges is a picture of the rational or reasonable dental patient: specifically afraid of those aspects of the situation that do in fact hurt, bothered and annoyed by those aspects that create discomfort, tolerant of those aspects that do not directly cause pain or discomfort, and clearly able to discriminate between the various categories. This ability to separate the pain inducers from the discomfort inducers, and in turn to separate these from the general background stands in marked contrast to the stereotype of the dental patient overwhelmed by general anxiety that expresses itself as undifferentiated aversion to all or most aspects of the treatment process, including the dentist. The stereotype has its theoretic origins in both the psychoanalytic and classic learning models, as these theories imply that traumatic or even "ordinary" fear will generalize from the particular source of the fear to surrounding objects and events. However, the data presented in Table 6.4 provide no support for the existence of a general dental-aversion syndrome, and this finding (which was predicted) paved the way for a detailed analysis aimed at further substantiating the hypothesis of the reasonable dental patient.

The Anatomy of Dental Anxiety

The data from the 25-item "Attitudes to Dental Treatment" questionnaire were submitted to a factor analysis. Factor analysis is a technique that examines the relationship between the statements in a questionnaire and identifies any natural groupings among the items. These groupings are called factors, and each factor summarizes a large number of related responses. Those individual attitudes that cluster together can then be described in structural terms, just as in biology individual cells that form part of a wider system develop their own particular structure.

Operationally factor analysis is based on the technique of correlation. Individual items will fall into a cluster if a majority of the subjects respond to the items in a similar fashion. For example, hypothetical items A, B, and C will emerge as a factor if those subjects that give a high response to item A also give high responses to items B and C, while those subjects that give a low response to item A, also give low responses to items B and C. The most useful factors are those that discriminate sharply among the subjects. Thus rather than merely saying that Subject X has a higher score on any one particular question than Subject Y, the information provided by factor analysis allows us to say that Subject X scores higher than Subject Y on a whole range of related questions, a much more useful assertion. Factor analysis therefore, is a means of reducing and simplifying a mass of items, providing that they all converge on the same underlying attitudinal structures.

The results of the factor analysis are presented in Table 6.5. The first point to note is that no general factor emerged. This means that no general attitude toward dental treatment was found, and contradicts assertions regarding the existence of a general dental-fear or dental-phobia syndrome. Rather, the

Table 6.5. Factor Analysis of "Attitudes to Dental Treatment" Questionnaire

Factor I (Discomfort)		Factor II (Pain)	
Statements*	Loading	Statements*	Loading
12. Keep mouth open	.71	10. Dentist drills on tooth	.82
20. Not being able to swallow	.70	25. Sound of drill	.76
		4. Needles and injections	.68
11. Water run in mouth	.66	13. Dentist picks at tooth	.61
21. Cotton wool in mouth	.58	17. Unable to stop dentist when it hurts	.56
9. Unable to move or talk	.56		
18. Room too hot or cold	.54		
6. Air or suction pump in mouth	.52		

*The numbers refer to the statment's original position in the "Attitudes to Dental Treatment" questionnaire.

analysis revealed the existence of two major clusters or factors. Table 6.5 presents the respective statements that make up each factor. Not all 25 items appear in the table; it is usual for the sake of simplicity, to include only items that load .5 or higher as defining a factor and statements loading less than .5 have therefore not been listed in the table. These latter statements were not clearly identified as belonging to either factor, nor did these items form a separate cluster of their own, and they are therefore not being considered in this section of the report.

The naming or labeling of factors is to some extent an arbitrary matter. Factor I has been labeled as a discomfort factor, and Factor II a pain factor. The pattern in the data closely parallels the results presented earlier, that anxiety varies with different aspects of the treatment situation. The present analysis confirmed that patients clearly distinguish between those aspects that produce pain and those aspects that result in discomfort.

Dental Anxiety as a Function of Type-of-Practice, SES, and Gender

The emergence of two separate factors on the 25-item "Attitudes to Dental Treatment" questionnaire permitted the data to be reduced and expressed in terms of the two factors. The technical operation consists of assigning factor scores to each subject. The 25 scores of each individual were transformed into two scores, one representing his or her level of experienced discomfort, and the second score representing his or her experienced pain. Each of these sets of scores were then submitted to an overall analysis of variance, to indicate what effect, if any, type-of-practice, SES, and gender of patients had on levels of discomfort and pain respectively. Analysis of variance is a technique that can reveal in one operation any "main" effects due to the respective

Table 6.6. Mean Factor I (Discomfort) Scores in Each Condition*

| SES | Type of Practice | | | | |
| | Preventive | | Restorative | | |
	Males	Females	Males	Females	Total
High	−.16	−.18	−.02	−.11	−.12
Low	+.13	+.27	−.10	+.18	+.12
Total	+.01		−.01		0
Total Males	= −.04				
Total Females	= +.04				

*A high score indicates high discomfort.

Table 6.7. Analysis of Variance of Factor I (Discomfort) Scores

Source	Sum of squares	DF	Mean square	F
Main effects	8.326	3	2.775	2.805
SES	7.449	1	7.449	7.530*
Practice	.149	1	.149	.151
Gender	.750	1	.750	.758
2-Way interactions	5.130	3	1.710	1.728
SES × Practice	2.591	1	2.591	2.619
SES × Gender	2.503	1	2.503	2.530
Practice × Gender	.051	1	.051	.051
3-Way interactions	.415	1	.415	.419
SES × Practice × Gender	.415	1	.415	.419
Explained	15.059	9	1.673	1.691
Residual	559.941	566	.989	
Total	575.00	575	1.000	

*p < .01

experimental conditions manipulated in the study, as well as any interaction effects that these conditions produce in combination.

Discomfort

Table 6.6 presents mean factor scores in each experimental condition for Factor I (discomfort), and Table 6.7 presents the analysis of variance for these data.

The only significant effect was for SES, such that patients from surgeries in the low socioeconomic suburbs experienced (or were willing to express) greater discomfort than high SES patients.

Table 6.8. Mean Factor II (Pain) Scores in Each Condition*

SES	Type of Practice				
	Preventive		Restorative		
	Males	Females	Males	Females	Total
High	−.13	+.14	+.10	+.20	+.08
Low	−.16	−.18	−.16	+.19	−.08
Total	−.08		+.08		0
Total Males = −.09					
Total Females = +.09					

*A high score indicates high pain.

Table 6.9. Analysis of Variance of Factor II (Pain) Scores

Source	Sum of squares	DF	Mean square	F
Main effects	14.524	3	4.841	5.018
SES	7.084	1	7.084	7.342*
Practice	3.494	1	3.494	3.621†
Gender	3.814	1	3.814	3.953‡
2-Way interactions	.772	3	.257	.267
SES × Practice	.290	1	.290	.301
SES × Gender	.039	1	.039	.040
Practice × Gender	.443	1	.443	.459
3-Way interactions	2.793	1	2.793	2.895
SES × Practice × Gender	2.793	1	2.793	2.895
Explained	28.878	9	3.209	3.325
Residual	546.122	566	.965	
Total	575.00	575	1.000	

*$p < .01$
†$p < .06$
‡$p < .05$

Pain

Table 6.8 presents mean factor scores in each experimental condition for Factor II (pain), and Table 6.9 presents the analysis of variance for these data.

The analysis revealed one large and highly significant effect, and two effects whose statistical significance is borderline. The large effect was due to SES, and unlike the results on discomfort, the evidence indicates that high SES patients experienced and/or are willing to admit to more pain than low

SES patients. The two smaller effects were due to type-of-practice and gender of patients: a) respondents in restorative practices experienced more pain than patients in preventive practices, and b) females experienced more pain than males.

The data indicate a complex relationship between the two components of dental anxiety and patient characteristics. The results seem to suggest that working-class patients are more sensitive to the discomfort of dental treatment, whereas middle class patients are more sensitive to pain, or are more willing to admit that they are experiencing pain. The more stoic attitude of the working-class patient to pain is certainly consistent with popular stereotypes, as is the notion that middle-class persons are more inhibited about making a fuss concerning relatively unimportant matters. However, the explanation is undoubtedly much more complex and an attempt to elucidate these findings appears in the next section, together with further empiric evidence concerning this issue.

The finding that females experienced (or were willing to admit to) more pain cannot be interpreted in isolation, but must be viewed against the general literature on individual differences in pain sensitivity. This literature was reviewed in Chapter 3 and is consistent with the finding that female dental patients experienced (or were willing to admit to) more pain than male patients.

The finding that preventive patients subjectively experienced less pain than restorative patients was predicted and confirms that the general social context of dental treatment significantly influences how patients respond. Thus patients in preventive surgeries are more likely to know and have a personal relationship with their dentist. It can be hypothesized that as personal contact between the dentist and a patient increases, the patient's confidence in the dentist's ability will increase, the patient will feel less anxious, and there will also be a decrease in the amount of pain experienced. An alternate explanation for the finding that preventive patients experience less pain may be that preventive dentistry is veridically less painful than restorative dentistry.

To test the hypothesis that patient confidence is systematically related to the social psychology of the dental treatment situation, a special questionnaire measuring patients' confidence in their dentist was included in the study, and these data will now be presented.

Patients' Confidence in Their Dentist

Patients' confidence in their dentist was measured by means of a six-item scale reproduced below. The responses to the six items were added up for each subject, producing a general confidence score, with a high value indicating high confidence.

CONFIDENCE SCALE

1. How *confident* do you feel about what your dentist is doing when he or she is working on your teeth?

   Not at all confident : 1 : 2 : 3 : 4 : 5 : Extremely confident

2. How *effective* do you think a dentist can be in *preventing* further dental disease?

   Not at all confident : 1 : 2 : 3 : 4 : 5 : Extremely confident

3. How *confident* do you feel about what your dentist tells you about your teeth?

   Not at all confident : 1 : 2 : 3 : 4 : 5 : Extremely confident

4. How *effective* do you think a dentist can be in restoring decayed or damaged teeth?

   Not at all confident : 1 : 2 : 3 : 4 : 5 : Extremely confident

5. How *competent* do you think your dentist is in general?

   Not at all confident : 1 : 2 : 3 : 4 : 5 : Extremely confident

6. How *confident* do you feel about your dentist in general?

   Not at all confident : 1 : 2 : 3 : 4 : 5 : Extremely confident

Table 6.10 presents the mean amount of confidence expressed in each of the experimental conditions, and Table 6.11 presents the analysis of variance for these data.

The analysis confirmed that: a) patients in preventive surgeries expressed more confidence in their dentists than patients in restorative surgeries, b) high SES patients expressed more confidence than low SES patients, and c) female patients expressed more confidence than male patients. Finally, an internal analysis using age as a covariate revealed a strong positive relationship between age and confidence, that is, the older the patient, the more confidence he or she expressed.

The confidence data are consistent with, and help to explain the findings

Table 6.10. Mean Confidence Scores in Each Condition*

| SES | Type of Practice | | | | |
| | Preventive | | Restorative | | |
	Males	Females	Males	Females	Total
High	27.33	27.78	25.79	27.02	26.97
Low	25.69	26.63	24.78	25.97	25.73
Total	26.83		25.88		26.37
Total Males	= 25.89				
Total Females	= 26.85				

*A high score indicates high confidence.

Table 6.11. Analysis of Variance of Confidence Scores

Source	Sum of squares	DF	Mean square	F
Main effects	348.962	3	116.321	7.872
SES	77.962	1	77.962	5.276*
Practice	107.383	1	107.383	7.268†
Gender	161.656	1	161.656	10.941‡
2-Way interactions	8.448	3	2.816	.191
SES × Practice	.289	1	.289	.020
SES × Gender	2.567	1	2.567	.174
Practice × Gender	5.593	1	5.593	.378
3-Way interactions	4.388	1	4.388	.297
SES × Practice × Gender	4.388	1	4.388	.297
Explained	1097.706	9	121.967	8.255
Residual	8363.042	566	14.776	
Total	9460.748	575	16.453	

‡$p < .001$
†$p < .01$
*$p < .05$

on patient anxiety. There is a strong indication that patient confidence mediates anxiety. Overall, preventive patients are more confident, and again overall, they experience less pain than restorative patients. However this relationship is influenced by other interacting effects. In particular, the tendency for high SES patients to have greater confidence in their dentists appears to be cancelled out by their greater susceptibility to pain relative to low SES patients. In other words, high confidence by itself can only reduce but not overcome patient sensitivity to the painful aspects of dental treatment, but probably explains why high SES patients experience less discomfort (Factor I) than low SES patients.

In addition to patient confidence, two other patient characteristics can be expected to have an effect on how the dental situation is perceived. These are the stereotypes that patients hold about their dentists, and the degree of accurate knowledge patients possess about dental health and care. These two variables were also systematically explored in the present study.

Patients' Stereotypes About Their Dentist

Psychologists use the concept of a stereotype to refer to "pictures in the mind" (Allport, 1958; Katz and Braly, 1933, 1935; Klineberg, 1966) or generalized attitudes that individuals hold about other persons or classes of persons. Stereotypes can be more or less veridical, and most contain at least a "kernel of truth" (Campbell, 1967). Stereotypes can be positive or negative—the target can be perceived either more or less favorably than is objectively the case, but most of the literature has been concerned with negative stereotypes. For practical purposes, the veridicality of a stereotype is irrelevant, as people will respond to others in terms of their perceptions of the others' characteristics, rather than the others' objective qualities. Stereotypes are very resistant to modification.

The stereotypes that patients hold about their dentists were measured by means of a "belief" questionnaire, which is reproduced below. All the items imply a negative attitude toward or perception of the dentist. The questionnaire was scored by adding up the number of items endorsed (ticked) by the respondent, so that the higher the score, the more negative the stereotype.

BELIEF QUESTIONNAIRE

1. Which of these do you believe to be true of your dentist? Tick as many or as few (or none) of the following:

_____X-rays are taken too often

_____Sometimes is careless

_____The dentist tries to make you come to too many appointments

_____Needles are given too frequently

_____Needles are not given enough

_____The dentist only creates more problems when you go and see him or her so that you have to go and see them again (example: making a hole in one tooth while the dentist is supposed to be filling another)

_____Write in any others _____

_____

_____

2. Which of these do you believe to be true of your dentist? Tick as many or as few (or none) of the following:

_____The dentist does not explain why or what he or she is doing

_____The dentist does not give you time to explain what you think is wrong.

_____The dentist does not give you time to ask questions

_____The dentist charges too much

_____All too often the dentist tells you it is not going to hurt when he knows it will.

_____The dentist does not give you enough dental health education

_____The dentist asks questions when your mouth is full of fingers or instruments so that you can not answer

_____There is too much chatter about everything but your teeth

_____The dentist is too impersonal

_____Write in any other _____

_____

_____

Table 6.12 presents the mean number of stereotypes held in each of the experimental conditions and Table 6.13 presents the analysis of variance for these data. The results indicate that patients in the restorative surgeries held significantly more negative stereotypes of their dentists than patients in preventive surgeries, and that males were more negative than females. An internal analysis using age as a covariate revealed that the older the patient, the more positive were his or her perceptions of the dentist. Finally, the absolute level of stereotyping was low in all the conditions, the largest mean being 1.94 in the Restorative Male Low SES condition.

The stereotype data parallel and corroborate the results on patient con-

Table 6.12. Mean Number of Stereotypes in Each Condition*

SES	Type of Practice				
	Preventive		Restorative		
	Males	Females	Males	Females	Total
High	1.17	0.72	1.57	1.04	1.13
Low	1.10	1.04	1.94	1.14	1.31
Total	1.01		1.43		1.22
Total Males	= 1.45				
Total Females	= 0.99				

*A high score indicates more negative stereotypes.

Table 6.13. Analysis of Variance of Stereotype Scores

Source	Sum of squares	DF	Mean square	F
Main effects	56.486	3	18.829	6.995
SES	.425	1	.425	.158
Practice	23.565	1	23.565	8.754*
Gender	32.213	1	32.213	11.967†
2-Way interactions	7.700	3	2.567	.954
SES × Practice	1.640	1	1.640	.609
SES × Gender	.036	1	.036	.013
Practice × Gender	6.028	1	6.028	2.239
3-Way interactions	3.722	1	3.722	1.383
SES × Practice × Gender	3.722	1	3.722	1.383
Explained	113.707	9	12.634	4.693
Residual	1523.598	566	2.692	
Total	1637.306	575	2.847	

†$p < .001$
*$p < .01$

fidence in regard to the important variable of type-of-practice: preventive patients are not only more confident about their dentists than restorative patients, but they also hold fewer negative stereotypes. The stereotype findings are also consistent in the case of the sex variable (females are more confident and hold fewer stereotypes than males), and age (the older the patients, the more confident they are and the fewer stereotypes they hold).

To obtain a description of what annoyed patients the most about their dentists, a frequency distribution of the complaints was prepared and these data appear in Table 6.14. The most frequent complaint was "The dentist charges too much," endorsed by 157 (27%) of the subjects, closely followed by "The dentist asks questions when your mouth is full of fingers or instruments so that you cannot answer." These data confirm the view of the "rational" patient. Only seven out of the 576 respondents (a little over 1%) felt that dentists created more problems, and only 10 patients (1.7%) complained that needles are not given enough. However, 27% of the subjects complained about the cost, 26% felt annoyed about being asked questions at

Table 6.14. Frequency Distribution of Complaints

Statements	Number and percentage of subjects endorsing each statement	
1. The dentist charges too much	157	27%
2. The dentist asks questions when your mouth is full of fingers or instruments so that you cannot answer	148	26%
3. The dentist does not explain why or what he or she is doing	53	9%
4. The dentist does not give you time to ask questions	52	9%
5. X-rays are taken too often	50	9%
6. The dentist does not give you enough dental health education	49	8%
7. All too often the dentist tells you it is not going to hurt when he knows it will	38	7%
8. The dentist tries to make you come to too many appointments	32	6%
9. Needles are given too frequently	25	4%
10. The dentist does not give you time to explain what you think is wrong	25	4%
11. Sometimes is careless	21	4%
12. The dentist is too impersonal	18	3%
13. There is too much chatter about everything but your teeth	15	3%
14. Needles are not given enough	10	2%
15. The dentist only creates more problems when you go and see him or her so that you have to go and see them again (example: making a hole in one tooth while the dentist is supposed to be filling another)	7	1%

the wrong time, and a significant proportion were concerned about the effect of x-rays (50 or 9%), insufficient explanation of the procedure (53 or 9%), insufficient time (52 or 9%), and insufficient dental health education (49 or 8%). The figures are all the more notable given the reluctance of patients to openly criticize their dentists, and it is likely that these stereotypes are much more widely held than the raw data indicate.

Patients' Knowledge About Dental Health and Care

The amount of accurate information about dental care was measured by means of a "Dental Knowledge Questionnaire", which is reproduced below. The questionnaire was scored by awarding two points for each item that had a perfect answer, and one point for an item with a partially correct answer. The total score reflected the patient's knowledge about dental care; the high-

DENTAL KNOWLEDGE QUESTIONNAIRE

1. Name one thing that you think is a main cause of tooth decay:
   _____

2. Name the one most effective thing that you think you can actively do to prevent tooth decay:
   _____

3. Name one thing that you think is the main cause of gum disease:
   _____

4. Name the one most effective thing you think your dentist can do to help preserve oral health:
   _____

5. What is dental plaque?
   _____

6. What do you think is the one most important thing your dentist has taught you about dental care:
   _____

7. Which of the following do you think is the best type of tooth brush? Place at least one tick in each column.

   [___] soft bristle   [___] small head

   [___] medium bristle   [___] medium head

   [___] hard bristle   [___] large head
   _____

8. What do you consider to be the best way to clean your teeth?
   _____

er the score the more extensive and accurate the patient's information. Table 6.15 presents the mean knowledge scores in each of the experimental conditions and Table 6.16 presents the analysis of variance for these data. The results reveal large and significant differences in the knowledge domain for all three variables. Thus preventive patients are much better informed than restorative patients, high SES patients are better informed than low SES patients, and females are better informed than males. These data corroborate the stereotype, confidence, and anxiety findings, and indicate the importance of dental health education. Preventive patients are better informed, more confident, hold fewer negative stereotypes, and experience less pain than re-

Table 6.15. Mean Knowledge Scores in Each Condition*

| SES | Type of Practice | | | | |
| | Preventive | | Restorative | | |
	Males	Females	Males	Females	Total
High	10.78	11.39	6.69	8.47	9.33
Low	10.13	10.33	6.29	6.28	8.25
Total		10.65		6.93	8.80
Total Males = 8.47					
Total Females = 9.12					

*A high score indicates greater knowledge.

Table 6.16. Analysis of Variance of Knowledge Scores

Source	Sum of squares	DF	Mean square	F
Main effects	2192.361	3	730.787	63.334
SES	178.748	1	178.748	15.491†
Practice	1952.197	1	1952.197	169.187†
Gender	64.549	1	64.549	5.594*
2-Way interactions	56.968	3	18.989	1.646
SES × Practice	4.012	1	4.012	.348
SES × Gender	46.570	1	46.570	4.036
Practice × Gender	6.293	1	6.293	.545
3-Way interactions	18.460	1	18.460	1.600
SES × Practice × Gender	18.460	1	18.460	1.600
Explained	2370.938	9	263.438	22.831
Residual	6530.889	566	11.539	
Total	8901.826	575	15.481	

†$p < .001$
*$p < .02$

storative patients. The same consistent pattern was obtained in the case of gender classification: females are better informed, more confident, and hold fewer negative stereotypes than males. The pattern is repeated when the data are classified by SES: high SES patients are better informed and more confident than low SES patients.

The knowledge and confidence variables are the two factors that appear as significant effects in each of the three experimental conditions (type-of-practice, SES, and gender). Knowledge and confidence must therefore be regarded as cornerstones in the overall patient-dentist relationship. There is considerable evidence in social psychology that the knowledge a person possesses in a particular domain provides the foundation for the attitudes he or she holds in that area (Festinger, 1957). Although the present study produced no direct evidence that knowledge plays a primary role in the dental domain, the overall pattern in the data supports the following extrapolation from the general literature on attitude formation: the amount of accurate knowledge that patients possess about dentistry will systematically affect their perception of the dentist, their confidence in the dentist, their degree of anxiety arousal in the dental situation, and the amount of pain they experience. Although these variables are interrelated so that each complexly affects all the others, the cognitive (knowledge) component undoubtedly acts as a pivot for the whole system. It is also the domain most accessible to intervention.

Summary and Conclusions

The study produced three sets of results. The first finding was that patients discriminate between two aspects of the dental situation, namely those aspects that are painful, and those aspects that are uncomfortable. The painful aspects arouse fear and anxiety, whereas the uncomfortable aspects of dental treatment arouse annoyance. These findings supported the hypothesis that the majority of patients are entirely rational in their approach to dental treatment. The results do not support the psychoanalytic model of dental anxiety as an inevitable and largely unconscious reaction to oral intrusion. The results also do not support the learning theory model of dental anxiety as nonspecific fear, initially attached to actual pain producing agents but subsequently generalized to all aspects of the dental situation. Instead, the data unequivocally confirm that patients make a distinction between the various elements of dental treatment and respond to each element rationally and appropriately.

The second set of results pertained to the detailed analysis of the effect of several social and psychologic variables on how patients responded to the dental situation. The antecedent or independent variables were concerned with who the patients were, their occupation, gender and age, and the type of practice they attended. The outcome or dependent variables were concerned with the patients' reactions, perceptions, and attitudes, and included patients' ratings of confidence, stereotypes about their dentists, and their knowledge of dental hygiene. These results have been summarized in Table 6.17. The significant relationships are indicated by an X in the respective cell.

All the relationships in Table 6.17 form a coherent pattern. Thus preventive patients are better informed, hold fewer negative stereotypes and are more confident; higher SES patients are better informed and more confident; females are better informed, hold fewer negative stereotypes, and are more confident; and older patients are more confident and hold fewer negative stereotypes. These data conclusively establish the existence of a systematic pattern of relationships among: a) the *cognitive* variable of accurate knowledge about dental hygiene, b) the *perceptual* variable of negatively stereotyping the dentist in the absence of such accurate knowledge, and c) the *affective* variable of confidence as a function of what the patients know about dental procedures, what they believe about their dentist, and how they perceive the dentist. These relationships constitute the social psychology of the dentist-patient system.

The third set of results pertains to relating the social psychology of the dentist-patient situation to dental anxiety. The anxiety results have been summarized in Table 6.18. The significant relationships are indicated by an X in the respective cell. Reading Table 6.18 in conjunction with Table 6.17

Table 6.17. The Social Psychology of the Dental Situation: Summary of Results*

Independent variables	Higher confidence	Fewer stereotypes	Greater knowledge
Preventive Practice	X	X	X
Higher SES	X		X
Females	X	X	X
Older Patients	X	X	

*An X indicates a significant relationship between the two variables.

Table 6.18. Dental Anxiety: Summary of Results*

	Type of anxiety	
Independent variables	Less discomfort	Less pain
Preventive Practice		X
Higher SES	X	
Lower SES		X
Males		X

*An X indicates a significant relationship between the two variables.

shows that the type-of-practice variable produced a consistent effect across both the social-psychologic and the anxiety domains: preventive patients were more confident, held fewer stereotypes, possessed greater accurate knowledge, *and* experienced less pain than restorative patients. Such consistency is partially lacking in the SES category, and absent in the gender classification. Higher SES patients have more confidence and knowledge *and* experience less discomfort, but feel more pain than low SES patients. This inconsistency may be attributed to a less stoic attitude to pain by the middle class, possibly related to the more sedentary life-style of persons in nonmanual occupations.

The inconsistency is even more pronounced in the data on gender differences. Although females have greater confidence and knowledge and harbor fewer negative stereotypes, they nevertheless experience more pain than males. This finding points to a fundamental problem in any research connected with the experience of and tolerance for pain. As we saw in Chapter 3, pain tolerance is complexly determined by at least five sets of conditions: (1) individual genetic dispositions (presumably these were randomly distributed in the study); (2) individual differences related to past experience with painful stimuli (also presumably randomly distributed in the study); (3) biologically related categories such as gender and age (gender was systematically varied and age measured in the study); (4) broad systematic environmental, physical-ecologic, and social-psychologic factors associated with a person's life style, such as his or her occupation, income, and cultural and ethnic identity (SES was systematically varied and culture controlled in the study); and (5) the contemporary social-psychologic context of the interaction, including the quality of the relationship (this was systematically varied in the study through the type-of-practice manipulation). These variables combine complexly to determine the degree of pain tolerance, and, depending on the constellation, may have either an additive or averaging influence, that is, either increase the prevailing effect or cancel each other out.

Implications for the Management of the Dental Situation

A major implication of the present study is to concentrate on those conditions that are amenable to change. Thus dentists can do very little about the SES or gender of the patients, but should be aware that high SES and female patients are likely to have a lower pain threshold, and use that knowledge accordingly. There is also very little that the dentist can do about further reducing the aversive consequences of those procedures that most patients consider to be painful (identified in the present study as the pain fear factor), short of administering a general anesthetic. However, it may be feasible to reduce many of the aversive consequences of those procedures that create annoyance (identified in the present study as the discomfort factor). Further research is needed to systematically explore the management of these procedures because most of them are in principle capable of being modified.

Finally, there is a great deal that individual dentists and the profession generally can do about improving the social psychology of the dentist-patient relationship. The evidence implies that dentists should adopt more explicitly the role of dental health educators. Further research is needed to establish the parameters of the role of the dental health educator. In particular, the hypothesis should be tested that the dentist-patient relationship would be enhanced if education were to become a more central part of the consultation. At present, education is typically conducted for a brief period only, often at the end of the consultation when the patient may not be in the right frame of mind or body to absorb much knowledge. The present study confirms other surveys reviewed elsewhere in this book that overall, patients are not very well informed about dental hygiene, suggesting that current methods of education are not sufficient to impart accurate knowledge about relatively simple matters, nor is what is being done now enough to dispel negative stereotypes. It is realized that there are serious practical problems in devoting precious consultation time to education. Perhaps one solution may be for the dentist to conduct occasional group sessions, at a nominal cost, devoted solely to education, which all patients are urged to attend. It may also be possible to produce a video tape about dental hygiene and play this film through video monitors in the waiting room. A further possibility would be to enlarge the role of the dental nurse to include dental education and arrange for the nurse or receptionist to conduct live demonstrations of dental hygiene in the waiting room.

A related hypothesis is that the dentist-patient relationship would be enhanced if the dentist were to adopt more explicitly the role of manager of the long-term dental health of the patient. This hypothesis is implied by the data on the more positive attitudes of preventive relative to restorative patients, and by evidence that accurate knowledge mediates greater confidence and lower stereotyping. In particular, the prediction should be tested that dentists who are seen as promoting the continuing dental health of the patient will inspire greater confidence and be the target for fewer negative perceptions, than dentists who merely concentrate on the contemporary problem of restoring the patient's teeth.

A major obstacle in the way of enlarging the dentist's role so as to include the educational and "pastoral" functions, is the relative infrequency of visits. It is very difficult for a personal relationship to develop between individuals who only see each other at annual or even six-month intervals. This suggests the hypothesis that all three problems (how to educate effectively, how to function effectively in a long-term preventive capacity, and how to personalize the relationship) could be ameliorated by interspersing conventional dental consultations with sessions devoted purely to educational aims, perhaps conducted in small groups. This would increase the frequency of dentist-patient contact to perhaps four or six occasions annually, and also have the important side effect of the patient and the dentist interacting under conditions where neither person was under stress.

In summary, four implications for the management of the dental situation have emerged from the present study:

1. to modify the discomfort-producing aspects of treatment so that patients experience less annoyance;
2. to devote more resources and consultation time to education;
3. to place greater emphasis on long term management;
4. to have more frequent contact between the dentist and patient.

7
Community-Based Dental Health Education

Stimulating the Demand for Preventive Dental Care

Increasingly, public health authorities in a variety of countries are trying to raise the level of community dental health. In practice this means trying to change existing attitudes and behavior and/or instilling new attitudes and behaviors, particularly those that will prevent or minimize the occurrence of dental decay. Changing attitudes and behavior are central topics in social psychology and a great deal of empiric research and theory building about these processes has accumulated over the past 80 years. It is outside the scope of this book to provide a general review of this huge literature, nor would it be appropriate to do so. Rather, we propose to describe those theoretic models that have particular relevance to public health education and which have stimulated empiric research in this field. An important principle to be kept in mind is that public health education programs that are soundly based in theory are more likely to be effective than programs that do not have such a base.

Elsewhere in this book we reviewed studies that concentrated on developing particular dental health-generating habits such as toothbrushing, concluding that the active acquisition of skills is more effective than passive, information-based learning. Our concern in this section is to go beyond such specific processes and principles and take a broader, more general approach to health education. The aim will be to proceed from low-level theories such as the active learning principle referred to earlier accounting for the acquisition of habits, to medium-level theories such as the Health Belief model, which accounts for the development of more general cognitive and behavioral orientations, and finally, to a comprehensive model that takes into account the major personal and sociocultural forces that affect health-related behavior.

Low-Level Theories

Research in psychology has identified a number of principles that can be used to change or instill particular attitudes and behaviors. Many of these are derived from learning theory and are used in behavior modification programs. These principles were reviewed in Chapter 5, mainly from the perspective of reducing dental anxiety. However, some of the constructs can also be applied to stimulate preventive oral hygiene habits such as toothbrushing, the most relevant principles being reinforcement, practice, praise, and feedback or knowledge of results.

Social psychology also has generated a number of specific principles that can be used in the service of attitude change. One such method is peer group decision making, which has been found to be effective in changing the attitudes of motorists and presumably would work in other public health fields. The approach is based on the pioneering work of Lewin (1947) who established that attitudes, particularly in young people, are related to their need to be accepted by their peers. Consequently, persons will hold those attitudes that they consider to be valued by their peers. A great deal therefore depends on what the group norm is, or to be precise, what the perceived norm is, and how much a person wants to be accepted by the peer group. This has particular relevance for devising traffic safety education programs, especially for young people. In many groups the norm favors heavy drinking and fast, uninhibited driving. Injunctions, threats, and appeals by parents, police, or safety experts to change these practices are unlikely to be accepted because they would require an individual to became a deviant in the group. Thus the attitude will resist change because it fulfills an important function for the individual, that of gaining access to and being accepted by a valued group. There may well be parallels in the dental field, with children engaged in toothbrushing behavior being regarded as sissies.

The solution is to try and shift the attitudes of the whole group, to make groups rather than individuals the targets of an influence attempt. This was the strategy adopted by Clark and Powell (1984) in their work with young drivers. Men under the age of 25 years who had been in at least one accident, participated in the study. They attended three sessions to talk about their attitudes toward cars and driving, bringing their friends with them. Before the discussions began, attitude scales about driving and drinking were administered, using items such as: When you are driving, do you push your way through or wait your turn? Do you drink and drive?

The group discussions were conducted with the aim of getting the subjects to explore their own attitudes and behaviors rather than to moralize about them. In the third session the group was asked if they would like to come to some sort of decision about the things they had been discussing for the past two weeks. They were then given the attitude scales again. The results showed that their attitudes changed significantly in the desired direction. A control group that had not been exposed to group discussion, but only had their attitudes measured twice during the same three-week interval, showed no change in their scores. The study clearly demonstrates the effectiveness of using the group as a change agent. In particular, it shows that peers rather than outside experts and authority figures can be very effective in changing and maintaining desirable behaviors. The technique has obvious applications in the field of oral hygiene, but a search of the literature has not revealed a study that explicitly uses this approach.

Another change method stemming from social psychology is the forced-compliance paradigm (Festinger and Carlsmith, 1959). The basic idea is to induce subjects to comply with some request. The compliance is said to be "forced" in the sense that subjects would not normally wish to undertake the requested behavior. Consequently, subjects have to choose between refusing to comply and antagonizing the person making the request, or they must commit themselves to behaving in a way that they know to be inconsistent with their true feelings. This sets up an aversive state of cognitive dissonance (Festinger, 1957), which the subjects can reduce by changing their attitude to make it consistent with the behavior they have been drawn into. More generally, the forced-compliance paradigm implies that one way to change attitudes is to first induce the person to change the corresponding behavior, which is contrary to the accepted wisdom that attitude change must precede behavior change.

A number of studies have confirmed this effect (for a recent review, see Eiser, 1986), but the phenomenon is most easily produced in highly contrived laboratory settings. Still, one can think of ways in which the process might be put in the service of oral hygiene. Presumably, once people have been induced to engage in a slightly effortful task such as toothbrushing or flossing, they need to justify this behavior to themselves. One way of doing this may be to convince themselves that the practice has some utility. A scan of the literature has not revealed any study explicitly using this principle to promote oral hygiene. Cognitive dissonance theory and the forced-compliance paradigm have been applied to an analysis of pain. Bayer (1985) suggests that there are many times when patients may experience inducements to inaccurately report their pain. Patients may respond to social pressure to stoically bear their pain and therefore report less pain than they actually experience. At other times there may be inducements to exaggerate the level of pain or to persist in reporting it after it has been resolved. Presumably the level of felt or experienced pain is to some extent affected by the levels that patients are induced into reporting. Bayer produces no evidence for this effect, but it is certainly implied by the theory.

The attribution process (see an earlier discussion of this concept in Chapter 6) can also be put in the service of preventive health programs. For instance, as Eiser (1982) has pointed out, the concept of addiction, say to smoking, is very much bound up with how people explain their own and each other's behavior; or, more specifically, to what do they attribute the causes of their own and another's behavior. The same principle applies to any act that has health-related consequences.

A basic assumption of attribution theory is that people explain their own behavior differently from the way they explain the behavior of others—that there is a fundamental distinction between how *actors* and *observers* account for behavior. Jones and Nisbett (1971) have shown that when people are asked to account for their own behavior (actors), they tend to offer situational explanations, but when asked to explain the behavior of others, to assume the role of an observer, they tend to make attributions in terms of the internal, enduring personality characteristics of the other individual. To illustrate, if I am asked why I came late to a dinner party, I will probably answer that it was due to the taxi not turning up on time, or that the traffic was heavy, or that something unexpected came up at work that detained me, all genuine and not made-up stories. However, if asked why I thought some other person was late, I as an observer am likely to attribute the other's behavior to some enduring trait possessed by that individual, such as chronic tardiness, absent-mindedness, or social insensitivity.

According to Eiser (1982), this is exactly the pattern that smokers (actors) use to explain their own smoking, as compared with the explanations offered by nonsmokers (observers) to account for the behavior of smokers. Nonsmokers are much more likely to label the smoker as addicted (i.e., that their smoking is due to some enduring, internal characteristics of the person), than were smokers when asked to give reasons why they smoked. Nonsmokers also underestimated the amount of pleasure obtained by smokers, and the extent to which smokers were frightened about the risks to their health. In other words, in the view of the nonsmoker, the average smoker is addicted, does not obtain much pleasure from smoking, and is relatively unconcerned about any associated health risks. The apparent irrationality of smokers is explained by making the personal, simplistic attribution that smokers are "addicted", a circular argument about the alleged distinctive attributes of smokers. Not only does this fail to provide a genuine explanation for the behavior, it also tends to deflect attention from any possible situational conditions that might contribute to the maintenance of the habit. Smokers, however, when they analyze their own behavior, take a much more complex view. They are fully aware of the positive and negative properties of tobacco consumption, of the difficulties involved in stopping, and of the personal and social consequences of their "addiction."

The practical implication of an attributional analysis for designing preventive health programs is to move away from a personality-oriented explanation of the target behavior, to a more complex, situation-based one. To illustrate, characterizing persons who do not brush their teeth as slothful, lazy, and irresponsible is not very helpful. Even if this were true, it is difficult to see how construing the problem in this way could lead to a feasible solution of it, short of providing psychotherapy to those individuals with "weak" personalities. A situational attribution, on the other hand, which will explain poor oral hygiene behavior in terms of circumstances such as a lack of relevant knowledge—poor facilities and resources for carrying out preventive oral hygiene (e.g., no toothbrush and no convenient place to brush one's teeth), lack of social and institutional supports for preventive practices—can be quite readily translated into appropriate remedial interventions. Some of these situation-based remedies will be discussed later in this chapter.

Middle-Level Theories

The middle-level theories are characterized by the assumption that there is a degree of consistency between attitudes, beliefs, and behavior. Although this is not always the case (see Bochner, 1980 for a review of this issue), the relationship between these three components holds sufficiently to make it a useful basis for change programs. These models take the more conventional view that beliefs and attitudes must be changed (using whatever particular methods might be appropriate to the occasion) before behavior change can occur.

In Chapter 2 we described the Health Belief model, which has been used both to explain and also to stimulate preventive health behavior. To recapitulate, the model states that people are more likely to take preventive action if they believe that they are susceptible to the disease, if they believe that the disease may have serious consequences for them, if they believe that by taking action the disease can be prevented or made less serious, and if they believe that taking action would not be worse than contracting the disease itself. As we saw, research on the extent to which the health beliefs of patients determine their actual preventive behavior provided equivocal results. Some studies supported the model whereas others did not. It is possible that the reason for the failure of some of these programs was that they used inappropriate methods, that the campaigns relied too much on imparting cognitive, abstract information rather than using a more active approach. The problem is that the core idea of the model states that beliefs are crucial in determining behavior, and therefore almost by definition it is highly reliant on using a cognitive approach.

Another model of behavior change based on the assumed positive correlation between attitudes and action is Ajzen and Fishbein's (1980) theory of reasoned action, which has been applied to a wide range of behaviors including smoking (Fishbein, 1982), alcohol use, contraceptive use, mother's choice of infant feeding methods, and consumer behavior (for a recent review of this literature, see Eiser, 1986). The theory of reasoned action is usually presented by means of fairly daunting diagrams with arrows joining a multitude of boxes (e.g., Ajzen and Fishbein, 1980; Hoogstraten, de Haan, and Horst, 1985), but its basic ideas are quite straightforward and can be summarized by a series of propositions. 1) The core idea is that behavior is determined by intention. 2) Intention, in turn, is determined by two complexly interacting components; a) beliefs about the consequences of performing or not performing the target behavior, and b) beliefs about whether other people would approve or disapprove of performing the behavior. Both these components include an expectancy as well as a value element. Will this consequence be made more or less likely by my performance of this behavior, and how good or bad for me would such a consequence be? Will other people whose opinion I respect be more or less likely to approve of me if I perform this behavior, and how much do I value the approval of such people? These various elements are presumed to combine multiplicatively to predict intention, which in turn predicts behavior.

In practice, problems arise in the empiric measurement of the various belief elements and how these measures should be weighted and combined. But in principle these problems can be overcome by paying more attention to the empiric operations underlying the various concepts. In some respects the theory of reasoned action is similar to and overlaps with the Health Belief model. However, it differs in two significant respects. First, it explicitly distinguishes between expectancy and value effects in predicting behavioral intentions. Although these two elements are implied in the Health Belief model, they are not as clearly separated. Second, the theory of reasoned action explicitly distinguishes between attitudinal and normative predictors of intentions. Indeed, the normative elements are almost totally ignored by the Health Belief model. This is a serious omission, particularly in the field of health education, where it is important to distinguish between behaviors that may be performed because of the benefits the person expects to gain from it, and behaviors performed because the person wishes to gain the approval or avoid the disapproval of respected other people. The model can therefore explain why some people continue to engage in activities such as smoking or excessive drinking, which they know to be injurious to their health, but which they also know to be normative in their particular millieu. Thus, unlike the Health Belief model, the theory of reasoned action, because of its explicit social-psychologic orientation, would be quite capable of predicting the outcome of the earlier mentioned Clark and Powell (1984) study using the method of peer group discussion to change the attitudes of young car drivers.

A scan of the literature revealed one study that directly compared the efficacy of the theory of reasoned action with the Health Belief model to stimulate demand for dental care. Hoogstraten, de Haan, and Horst (1985) constructed three messages. One was based on the Ajzen and Fishbein (1980) model and stressed the positive consequences of seeking dental treatment and the advantages flowing from this. The second communication was based on the Health Belief model and stressed the subjects' susceptibility to dental disease, the consequences of bad dental hygiene, the possibility of losing teeth, the esthetic implications, and it was then pointed out that seeking dental treatment could prevent all this from happening. The third communication was based on the assumption that providing information on the subjects' rights to receive dental care would stimulate demand, and reminded them that as paid-up clients of an insurance company they should exercise their right to free or subsidized treatment.

The three messages were of similar length and format and were sent to insured clients of three Amsterdam insurance companies, who according to the records had not received regular dental treatment for at least two years. A control condition was also included in the study, in which clients received an application form for dental treatment only, without any message. The subjects were randomly assigned to the various conditions. The results showed that there were no significant differences among the three message conditions, and contrary to expectations, the response rate in the application-only condition exceeded that of the various experimental conditions. This experiment illustrates the difficulties associated with translating complex psychologic theories into practical grass-roots action. It seems that the mere provision of an application form acted as a sufficient trigger to seek dental treatment in this case. However, it should be remembered that the subjects were all paid-up clients of an insurance company, so that this result perhaps is not as surprising as it at first seems. Incidentally, the importance of "triggers" is predicted by the Health Belief model. Indirectly, therefore, the study provides some support for this theory, but because the manipulation of triggers was inadvertent, a valid conclusion about their theoretical significance cannot be drawn. The definitive experiment on the relative utility of the various psychologic models in constructing oral hygiene programs has yet to be conducted.

High-level theories

A comprehensive model would have to consider both within-skin (intra-psychic) as well as the between-skin (interpersonal) aspects of dental health education, and then go beyond these to relevant features of the sociopolitical context. The main advantage of such a model is to provide a checklist of the conditions that should be taken into account when planning a public dental health education program that takes place outside of the surgery.

Starting with the individual, the literature reviewed in this book indicates that about 15% of the general population is sufficiently anxious about dental treatment to avoid going to the dentist unless it becomes absolutely necessary. Any campaign wishing to reach this minority would have to take this into account and set up special programs aimed at identifying these individuals and then reducing their anxiety. Some of the available methods have been reviewed elsewhere in this book.

Next, it is necessary to consider the physical location where the program will take place and who the agents of change will be. This draws attention to what is sometimes forgotten, that successful programs will usually run their course in two parallel places, in a public or institutional setting, and also in the privacy of the home. Suitable institutions might be the school, place of employment, community health center, or other similar organization. This in turn raises the problem of gaining the active cooperation of those controlling these institutions. For instance, school teachers may regard dental health as outside their responsibility and perhaps even an intrusion on the time that they feel would be better spent on traditional academic topics. Employers may have the same attitude, feeling that it is not their role to foster public health. And sometimes peer attitudes may also not be particularly helpful. These sorts of barriers may prove to be the main stumbling blocks in setting up public dental health programs because people are unlikely to seek out professional advice on their own. However, they may (the operative word being "may") respond if the programs are brought to them.

Assuming that an institutional location has been secured, the next questions to ask are who the change agents will be, and what methods will be used? Will it be outside experts, teachers (if it is a school), the company nurse? Will the target be the individual or the peer group? Will the emphasis be on a cognitive approach to instill information and knowledge? Or will the aim be to impart relevant skills through behavior training, supported by rewards, reinforcements, praise, feedback, and knowledge of results? Will the purpose be to create appropriate norms and values about dental hygiene by establishing relevant beliefs about dental health? Or a combination of all these methods?

Finally, what environmental and institutional supports are there for the program? Is there a place where the participants can conveniently clean their teeth? Does the school vending machine or company canteen provide appropriate food and not stock harmful products such as sweets?

Even if the program has succeeded so far, the behaviors, skills, attitudes, beliefs, and values acquired in the school or work setting have to transfer readily to the home if they are to be maximally effective. This is probably the next major stumbling block to effective public dental health education. Because the parents and spouses of the children and workers did not directly participate in the program, they may not be as enthusiastic about the idea of preventive dental health. This is a problem particularly in the case of children. The parent packs the school lunches, controls the diet at home, and has the power to reward, ignore, or obstruct toothbrushing, flossing, and other preventive procedures, including taking the child to the dentist for regular check-ups. With adults the spouse plays a similar, but to some extent diminished role. It is here, too, that economic considerations enter into the picture—"Should we spend the money on preventive dental care or on a new hall carpet?" Social support (or its absence) in the home, as at work, is a crucial but usually neglected ingredient in public health campaigns, whether the target behavior is smoking, drinking, dieting, exercise, or toothbrushing.

Finally, the sociopolitical context cannot be ignored. Dental health programs cost money and the allocation of resources for such a purpose has obvious political implications. Governments must choose between spending money on public health, education, defense, and so forth. Within the community health domain, further choices must be made between campaigns against smoking, alcohol abuse, vaccinations, prenatal care, venereal disease, and all the other competing public health problems. There may also be vested interests that can impede action in a particular area. The efforts of the tobacco companies to muddy the waters regarding the relationship between smoking and ill health is a case in point. In the present instance, one can imagine that the large confectionary manufacturers or the sugar industry may feel threatened if there was too much adverse publicity about the link between dental decay and sweets. And at a broader level still, there are cultural differences in attitudes to oral health, linked to differences in esthetic values. For instance, in the United States, possessing and keeping straight, white teeth is a highly desirable social asset, and parents are willing to commit large resources to preventive orthodontic treatment for their children. In other cultures, teeth do not have such a high esthetic or socially desirable status, the implication being that it would be easier to persuade politicians in the United States to fund public dental health campaigns than it would, say, in Australia, where there would be fewer votes in it.

It may be of interest to compare and contrast the classes of behavior that have a high public health profile. These include smoking, alcohol abuse, drug and substance abuse, reckless driving, poor diet, lack of exercise, and poor oral hygiene habits. All have long-term harmful effects; all are more or less preventable through action under the control and within the capabilities of most individuals; all lead to personal suffering, and are a public burden on indexes such as lost working hours, increased medical and hospital expenditure, increased crime, family disruption, pressure on social services, and so forth. Another feature that they share in common is the assumption that prevention is better than cure, and that an early start, preferably in children, is desirable, certainly in the case of oral health, exercise, and dietary habits.

We can now ask a series of questions about these socially undesirable habits. What triggers or induces these behaviors? What maintains them? What are the conditions that produce resistance to change? What are their long-term consequences? And finally, under what conditions can the undesirable behaviors be changed?

Looked at in this way, some major similarities and differences between dental hygiene and several of the other public health areas emerge. Smoking, drinking, drug and substance abuse, fast driving, and overeating are all activities that lead to pleasure, at least in the initial stages, and tend to be social activities through which the individual establishes or maintains a positive social identity (Tajfel, 1981). Not seeking dental treatment has an entirely different origin, stemming as it does from a wish to avoid pain, at least in the immediate short term. Avoiding exercise has a similar origin, being perceived by many people as a noxious, effortful activity to be indulged in as little as possible.

All of the activities on the list lead to long-term aversive consequences, but the seriousness varies. All but poor dental hygiene can and do lead to premature death, whether from cancer, lung disease, heart failure, AIDS, or traumatic accidents, the time lag varying from a few months as in the case of some drug abuse or persistent poor driving, to several decades in the case of poor diet or smoking. With dental neglect, the consequences are not as dramatic, but nevertheless the prospect of a toothless, painful middle age cannot be too pleasing. The issue of the severity of consequences is important, because as we saw, the various attitude change models all employ this construct in their procedures, reminding people of the bad things that will happen to them if they fail to comply with the recommendations.

Poor dental hygiene differs from the other behaviors in that there is no social support for it. Therefore it ought to be less resistant to change. All the other activities are embedded in ongoing group activities and are therefore highly resistant to change. But because of the greater seriousness of the consequences of smoking, drinking, fast driving, and so forth, both in terms of personal misery as well as public expense, these behaviors may under the right conditions respond more readily to health education, the gradual move away from smoking being a case in point. Nevertheless, in these areas people have to give up something they enjoy. With oral hygiene, people have to take on something they will not enjoy, and may dislike intensely. Because of the greater perceived seriousness of smoking, drinking, unsafe driving, substance abuse, poor diet, and lack of exercise, these issues are likely to attract more political attention and public funding than the relatively less acute but nevertheless still quite significant social problem of poor oral hygiene.

There is no doubt that psychologic principles can be usefully applied to promoting dental health education outside of the surgery. However, to date very few large-scale campaigns have explicitly used this knowledge in their design and implementation. Clearly, this is a fruitful field for greater cooperation between dentists, public health officials, and social scientists. But there are usually structural barriers to achieving such cooperation. Most interdisciplinary efforts fail because each group gives priority to its own professional and research interests, and is often somewhat ignorant about the other speciality. Evans (1982) describes one attempt to overcome this particular problem. Doctoral students in the Department of Psychology at the University of Houston did some of their training at the University of Texas Dental School. Joint research was conducted, which had to be of sufficient intrinsic interest so that the findings would contribute to social psychology apart from their relevance to dentistry. Thus the professional needs and aspirations of both groups were made to coincide. The point of all this is that to merely exhort different disciplines to cooperate for the good of humankind is of little use because such appeals usually fail. What is required is to set up programs and institutional structures that meet the basic aims of both groups.

Let us pursue this theme with a concrete example. Psychologists like to do research that not only solves some particular problem, but that also adds to the understanding of some basic psychologic process. For instance, psychologists are not just interested in persuading people to brush their teeth after meals, but may be more concerned with elucidating the general principles of attitude change. To study opinion change processes, subjects are needed. Most research psychologists use students to serve as subjects in their experiments, and have been rightly or wrongly criticized for basing their conclusions on a somewhat limited and atypical sample of human beings. Indeed, cynics have described psychology as the science of undergraduate behavior. Dentistry provides an ideal solution to this problem. For instance, if the research topic is attitude change, there is an unlimited supply of easily accessible "real" people from all walks of life who could serve in experiments in which there is an attempt to persuade them to see the dentist more frequently, brush their teeth after meals, eat less sweets, or whatever. These experiments can be designed so that on the one hand they will be able to confirm or disconfirm general theoretic principles about the attitude change process and thereby add to the psychologic literature in this area; and on the other hand actually increase the number of people attending surgery, flossing their teeth, or eating celery instead of sticky cakes, thereby raising the level of dental health in the community and providing increased job satisfaction for individual dental practitioners. One topic that has been studied in this way is whether fear-arousing communications are more or less effective in persuasion, a topic that has obvious "pure" as well as applied implications, and one that admirably lends itself to being studied in a dental context (for a recent review of this literature, see Sutton, 1982). An excellent case can therefore be made for the interdependence of the two disciplines, with cooperation leading to mutual benefits that can only be achieved through such joint action. Unfortunately in practice the situation is quite different. Dentists by and large are hesitant about allowing psychologists into their surgeries, just as doctors are (Pendleton and Bochner, 1980), for a variety of reasons, some justified, some not. And many psychologists are reluctant to engage in what they (erroneouly) perceive to be of necessity ad hoc, narrowly applied research, and are (erroneously) concerned about the alleged inevitability of diminished experimental control in field settings such as the dental surgery. The most practical way to overcome these misperceptions and reservations on both parts is at the training stage, but very few universities have set up joint schemes such as the one described by Evans (1982).

Summary

Community-based dental health education can be regarded as a branch of applied social psychology. Research in the psychology of attitudes has revealed a number of guidelines for designing campaigns to establish, change, and maintain desirable oral hygiene attitudes and habits.

A distinction was drawn between low-, middle-, and high-level theoretic principles of attitude change. Low-level theories provide the rationale for particular techniques of persuasion, such as group discussion, forced compliance, active versus passive learning, the use of praise, knowledge of results, and so forth; and who the agents of change should be, such as experts, authority figures, or peers. Middle-level theories provide the rationale for campaigns aimed at changing general oral health-related beliefs and values, based on the assumption that there is a high degree of consistency between attitudes, beliefs, values, and actions. Two theories were reviewed, the Health Belief model, and the theory of reasoned action. The former emphasizes the negative consequences of not taking preventive action and the positive consequences of treatment; the latter theory emphasizes the social psychology of preventive health in pointing out that the behavior of people is shaped by the groups to which they belong and whose membership they value. A basic finding of social psychology is that individuals act in such a way as to gain access to and win approval from groups to which they wish to belong and whose acceptance they seek, even if the behaviors are dangerous or injurious to their health. A good deal therefore depends on what the group norm is. Attempts at persuading people to change habits that the group values will fail because that would make the individual an outcast in that group, a fate far worse than even death, particularly for teenagers.

High-level theories provide a general framework for community-based dental health education in identifying the various personal, situational, and sociocultural elements that can either facilitate or hinder such programs. These include the two major behavior settings where the programs occur, the institutional and home settings respectively, each with its potential supports and barriers. Political considerations, vested interests in society, competing demands of different public health areas, the relative seriousness of dental versus other community health problems, and cultural differences in attitudes to dental neglect, are some of the other features that have to be taken into account.

The chapter ends with an analysis of the difficulties that have prevented greater cooperation between the dental profession and the social sciences. The point is made that a potentially mutually rewarding, symbiotic relationship between the two groups is feasible. There is no reason why psychologists should not be able to combine the twin aims of doing "pure" research into basic psychologic processes with applied research of interest to the dental profession. Indeed, such an approach would enhance the quality of both the "pure" and the applied product in that the conclusions drawn would be based on a much more representative sample of subjects, engaged in much more realistic and relevant experimental tasks. However, to achieve this interdisciplinary link, structural changes in the training programs of both professions may be necessary.

8

Common Sense and Patient Management: Implications for Practice, Training, and Research

As we saw in Chapter 6, the social psychology of the dentist-patient relationship is made up of a set of interlocking elements. The attitudes that patients have toward the treatment and the dentist depend on how they perceive the dentist and the confidence they have in their practitioner. These variables in turn affect the degree of pain and anxiety patients experience, the level of satisfaction with the service, the amount of knowledge they retain about dental hygiene, and the extent to which they comply with their dentist's instructions. What mediates all of these responses is the nature and quality of the relationship between the patient and the dentist. Because it is usually the dentist rather than the patient who is the one to establish the terms on which dental care is delivered, it is also the dentist who largely determines what form the dentist-patient relationship will take.

Models of the Dental Profession

Dentistry, like many of the other professions, can follow different models, each with its own consequences for the relationship between the dentist and the patient. For instance, dentistry can be regarded as a purely commercial enterprise (Ozar, 1985), dental care being a commodity that dentists sell and patients buy. On this basis, the interaction between the dentist and the patient would boil down to each trying to maximize their gain from the exchange. Thus dentists would decide what sort of dental care they will provide, not in relation to the need of a patient, but rather what services the patient is willing to pay for. Under the commercial model, patient need has only an indirect role in determining dental care, its main function being to motivate the patient to part with money for the sake of increased well-being or comfort. Dentists who openly acknowledge such an orientation justify it by arguing that this leads to competition with other dentists in areas such as pricing, the use of modern equipment and procedures, brighter and more comfortable surgeries, anything that will attract dental consumers to themselves, away from other dentists, and that all this is in the long-term interests of the dental consumer as well as the profession.

An alternate model is the guild model, where the profession and its role in society is dominant. Dentists with this orientation regard themselves primarily as under an obligation to cater to patients' needs, to provide relief from suffering, and to increase oral health through prevention and education. One consequence of this model is to heighten the distinction between the expert professional on the one hand, and the passive lay receiver of this treatment on the other, leading to a relationship that is unequal in status and highly paternalistic. Dentists who openly acknowledge such an orientation justify it on the grounds that they are engaged in a highly technical and skilled enterprise and that they alone know best what is good for the patient, and that the asymmetrical distribution of power and autonomy is in the long-term best interests of the patients as well as the profession.

Although no hard evidence on this issue is available, it is likely that most dental practices are run on a mixture of the commercial and guild models. In other words, most dentists are interested in making money, but also care about their patients' welfare, and try to do their job in such a way as to harmonize these two goals. However, there is indirect evidence, some of which was reviewed earlier in this book, that dentists do tend to treat their clients as cases rather than as patients, that is, as a technical problem to be treated, with the sufferer as the passive recipient of highly skilled treatment. One of the conclusions that can be drawn from the literature is that this approach leads to patient reactance, thus thwarting both the commercial and the professional/therapeutic aims of the dentist because patients may attend the surgery less frequently as customers and their oral hygiene also may suffer. Clearly a third model of the dentist-patient relationship is required, one that is more genuinely interactive, with each responding to the other in personal as well as role-specific terms, and where the dentist tries to involve the patient in the treatment procedure. Such a model is entirely compatible with both the commercial and service orientations of the profession, since it has been found to have an enhancing effect in each of these domains.

Dimensions of the Dentist-Patient Relationship

A review of the literature has revealed several dimensions along which the dentist-patient relationship can vary. One is the *personal-impersonal* dimension. Many dentists tend to treat their patients as cases rather than persons. Other dentists as a matter of policy become more or less personally involved with their patients. The evidence suggests that dentists who establish a personal, warm, caring relationship with their patients are perceived in a more favorable light and have a more positive impact on patient anxiety, knowledge, and compliance, than dentists who are technically competent but keep their distance from their patients.

Another dimension in the dentist-patient relationship is the extent to which the dentist adopts the role of *health educator*. Dentists who explicitly assume responsibility for the long-term oral well-being of their patients will tend to have a much more personal relationship with their patients than dentists engaged mainly in restorative work. Another variable, confounded to some extent with the distinction between preventive and restorative care, is the *frequency and regularity of contact*. Dentists and patients who meet each other regularly and frequently are much more likely to establish a personal relationship than when the encounters are intermittent. Dentists in group practices and those doing primarily restorative work will therefore have less opportunity to establish closer links with their patients. Finally, *the socioeconomic status of the patients* constitutes another major variable. Dentistry is an expensive service. The evidence indicates that less affluent patients attend surgery less frequently than the well-to-do. Low SES patients are therefore less likely to enter into preventive care, probably a false economy in the long run but perhaps unavoidable in the short term for this category of patient. Because most dentists are middle class in origin and orientation, they already have a problem in communicating with patients who do not share their assumptions and outlook on life. This gap is widened further by the tendency of lower SES patients not to opt for the kind of dental care that is more personal in nature.

The Communication Gap

The common factor in all of the dimensions of the patient-dentist relationship is the extent to which dentists are able and willing to communicate effectively with their patients. As we have seen, there are many ingredients in the dental situation that militate against the establishment of rapport between dentist and patient. Two conditions in particular have contributed to creating interpersonal distance. One is the lack of training that dentists receive in interpersonal communication skills. The other is the constraining nature of the conventional dental appointments schedule.

Interpersonal Skills Training

In an American study, O'Shea, Corah, and Ayer (1984) gave a questionnaire to 977 dentists in which respondents were asked to rate 25 possible stressors in terms of how stressful they found each in their current practice. They were also asked some general questions on stress. Seventy-five percent of the respondents said that dentistry was more stressful than other occupations (i.e., whether true or not, this is how they *perceived* their occupation). The stressors mentioned most frequently included "falling behind schedule," "striving for technical perfection," "causing pain or anxiety in patients," "cancelled or late appointments," and "lack of cooperation from patients in the chair."

In a survey of 150 dentists, Cooper, Mallinger, and Kahn (1980) found that the most stressful aspects of the job were "coping with difficult patients" and "trying to keep to a schedule." Also perceived as stressful, but to a much lesser degree, were "taking on too much work," "relating to auxiliary staff," and "fulfilling administrative duties." The authors conclude that the major sources of stress stem from the dentist's managerial role rather than from the technical aspects of the job. This is also the view of Kent (1983), who found that the most frequent problems cited in a survey of 56 dentists in Sheffield, England, was communicating with difficult patients, managing patient anxiety, and in motivating their patients to engage in better preventive care. These and other authors suggest that more time should be spent in dental school on teaching prospective practitioners managerial, organizational, and social skills.

It has been estimated that only 3% of the dental curriculum is devoted to interpersonal skills training. The successful practice of dentistry requires highly complex technical skills as well as a thorough grounding in the biologic sciences, and it is therefore not surprising that there is not much room in the curriculum for subjects seen as being peripheral to the main task. Introducing social science topics into an already crowded course is therefore likely to be met with resistance by both faculty and students. For instance, a course in communication skills is offered to all freshman dental students at the School of Dentistry at the University of Mississippi (Runyon and Cohen, 1979). The course consists of five three-hour sessions, attended by a class of 35 students. Although most of the students thought that the training was useful and relevant, and a post-test showed some improvement in the communication skills of the students, this program has obvious limitations and merely emphasizes the low priority given to human relations training in the dental curriculum. In any case, it is debatable whether the undergraduate phase is the most appropriate time to introduce students to the interpersonal dynamics of their discipline. The best learning occurs when there is a distinct perceived need. This certainly seems to be the view of Blandford and Dane (1981) in their discussion of how to structure continuing dental education. Dentists are likely to perceive their lack in interpersonal skills most acutely in their first year or two as independent practitioners. That would seem to be the appropriate time to undertake a systematic course in general interpersonal communication skills, followed by training specifically tailored to the dental situation. There already is a tradition for helping professionals to acquire various postgraduate qualifications as part of their career development and specialization, so there is no reason why the acquisition of a qualification in interpersonal skills should not follow the same pattern.

Social skills are not a genetically fixed aspect of personality, but can be taught, learned, and practiced. In reviewing the relevant literature. Furnham (1983) shows that a good deal of social skills training (SST) has been applied to various groups within the medical profession, including trainee doctors taking medical histories, general practitioners, occupational therapists, and nurses. However, it appears that very little SST has been done with dentists, although there is a demonstrated need for such training, the technology for it is available, and there is a model for it in the related field of medicine that would readily transfer to dentists.

An excellent review of the SST literature as it pertains to the doctor-patient relationship can be found in Maguire (1981). Many of the problems that physicians encounter appear to be similar to those faced by dentists. These include poor interviewing skills hindering the collection of relevant information, the excessive use of leading questions and unfamiliar jargon, failure to respond to cues given by patients about their concerns, cutting off patients' communications, and neglecting to pursue important psychologic and social aspects of the complaint. All these issues would have some application in the dental context.

Many general practitioners (physicians) were found to use few empathic statements, avoid eye contact, and not talk about personal issues. They ended their consultations poorly and paid little heed to any background psychologic issues. A number of studies have also shown that many physicians are poor at or reluctant to provide their patients with information about their condition and treatment. One consequence of this is that patients tend not to fully understand what their doctors say to them, leading to the startling finding that on average, 50% of patients fail to comply with medical advice and treatment. This, too, is a problem for dentistry, particularly in the implementation of preventive programs.

Most of these basic communication and social skills are easily acquired by most people lacking them. Nevertheless, many health professionals are inadequate in this regard, despite evidence that communication skills often affect the care that patients receive and weigh on the successful outcome (or otherwise) of the treatment. This latter point is sometimes disputed or dismissed as being irrelevant. Traditional medical and (probably) dental education takes the view that the task of the profession is to diagnose and treat disease. Social and psychologic problems merit less attention, both in the training of practitioners, and in how these practitioners treat their patients, because it is assumed that excessive "psychologizing" will distract the practitioner from dealing with the "real" problem, namely the presenting physical symptom. This view, which completely ignores the evidence, much of it reviewed in this book, about the complex relationship between psychologic and physical determinants of ill-health, has two consequences. One is to place an increasing emphasis on the technology of health care rather than on the psychology of the patients being treated. Second, proposals to teach communication skills and psychology to health professionals are likely to be resisted on the grounds that the curriculum is already overcrowded and if any additional time were made available it ought to be devoted to a more intense treatment of core topics such as anatomy or physiology. However, there is some evidence, as we have seen elsewhere in this book, that the pendulum may be swinging the other way, as an increasing number of health professionals become aware of the consequences of their poor interpersonal skills, not just with their patients but also on their own effectiveness as healers and on their job satisfaction.

The Dental Appointments Schedule

The delivery of dental care is very expensive, being both a capital and labor-intensive enterprise. The modern dental surgery contains much high-technology equipment that represents a considerable capital investment. Dentists are highly trained professionals who expect and deserve a reasonable standard of income. Most of the work cannot be delegated to ancilliary, less well-paid staff. Futhermore, in addition to the dentist, at least one other trained person, usually a nurse, attends the patient. Clearly under these circumstances every minute of an appointment has to be utilized effectively, and most dentists interpret this to mean that they should devote all of the time to technical procedures. Consequently, there tends to be very little personal conversation between the dentist and the patient. The traditional surgery resembles an assembly line. The patient is ushered into the surgery by a receptionist, told to sit in the chair, and within 30 seconds the procedures have commenced. There is then intensive activity for about half an hour, the dentist obviously preoccupied with the technical details of the intervention and not paying much heed to anything else. At the conclusion of the session, immediately after the last rinse, the patient is politely but firmly led out to make another appointment and/or pay the bill. A new patient is ushered in, and the cycle starts afresh.

The dental schedule is not conducive to the establishment of a personal relationship between dentist and patient. Nor is it an ideal setting for health education. The meetings are infrequent and both participants are tense and preoccupied when they do meet. By the end of a working day the patients must seem like a blur to the dentist, all merging into one another. From the patient's point of view the dentist's features are also indistinct, blurred by the lights and the mask worn by the dentist, the perception further dulled by the discomfort surrounding the encounter.

What is the solution? It would be unrealistic to expect dentists to devote half of the appointment to personal conversation and/or health education. In any case, as research reviewed earlier has shown, most patients tend to be somewhat anxious when in the chair, reducing their ability to listen to the dentist and respond appropriately. One possibility, briefly referred to earlier, would be for dentists to run separate health education sessions for groups of say 10 patients at a time. The patients would be charged for this service, but at a rate that would be minimal for each individual, the group paying whatever it cost the dentist to perform a routine service to a single patient. In these sessions dentists could give formal presentations followed by a discussion in which patients would be encouraged to express their feelings as well as seeking health-related information. The sessions would be informal, each group meeting at weekly intervals for three or four consecutive weeks. Suitable refreshments could be served to set the tone. The aim, clearly conveyed to the patients by the dentist, would be threefold: a) to break down the barrier between dentist and patient and set up the beginnings of a personal relationship; b) to disseminate health education information and techniques; and c) to give patients an opportunity to reveal and discuss their fears and anxieties and to give dentists an opportunity to discover what is in their patients' minds so that appropriate remedial action can be planned and taken.

The Anxious Patient

The evidence suggests that almost all patients experience an increase in anxiety while in the chair. Fortunately the vast majority of these patients are able to tolerate their anxiety, control their behavior, and feelings, and allow the treatment to proceed with a minimum of fuss. However, there is a substantial minority of individuals who for various reasons experience levels of dental anxiety that seriously affect their attendance and disrupt procedures when the patient can be induced into the surgery. What can be done to reduce the anxiety of these patients, and improve their management?

Psychoanalysis and Patient Management

The evidence and arguments presented in this book suggest that the psychoanalytic approach to patient management has very little utility. It may be the case that patients are not fully aware of the reasons for their feelings and anxieties, but even if this were so the dental surgery is not a very good setting for insight-oriented psychotherapy. The same reasons that militate against the establishment of a personal relationship between dentist and patient prevent the development of a psychotherapeutic one. There are other problems. As it may take four or five years to conclude a successful psychotherapy, and it takes four or five years to train a person in the art of clinical psychology, it is simply impractical to propose a psychoanalytic solution to dental anxiety in the dental surgery. If dental-aversive individuals wish to enter into psychotherapy on their own account with an analyst or clinical psychologist, that is certainly their right but it is not a service that a dentist can be expected to provide.

Psychoanalysis in the dental surgery is therefore impractical. The evidence also suggests that it would not be effective. Psychoanalysis as a therapeutic procedure does not have a very high success rate relative to other treatments (Erwin, 1980; Eysenck, 1966; Rachman, 1971), and in the specific instance of dental aversion is probably the least preferred method. Nevertheless, there is an element of truth in many of Freud's original propositions. Authority figures do remind us of our parents, not necessarily due to any complicated unconscious mental gymnastics but because for most of us our parents were our first mentors and disciplinarians. Women patients may become erotically aroused in the chair not due to some long forgotten oedipal conflict but because the dentist is a much more handsome and attentive man than their husband. Men may develop homosexual anxieties not because of their repressed desires but due to their intimate personal space being violated by another male. Common sense dictates that dentists should be aware of these problems, and deal with them in a reasonable manner. This means not looking for deep-seated hidden causes, but discussing with the patient what the immediate, overt problem might be, and then dealing with it accordingly.

Behavior Modification and Patient Management

The evidence indicates that behavior modification techniques are effective in reducing patient anxiety. Many of these techniques can be applied in the dental surgery without unduly prolonging the treatment or increasing its cost. However, behavior therapy is a relatively complex procedure that only properly trained individuals should engage in. Futhermore, it would be inadvisable to train individuals simply in the techniques without providing them with the theoretic background on which the procedures are based. There are two solutions to this problem. The first is for interested dentists to acquire this training, ideally after they have successfully mastered the interpersonal skills curriculum referred to earlier. The second is for a dentist to establish a connection with a psychologist trained in behavior modification and refer patients to that specialist. In either case the patients would be expected to pay for the additional treatment they receive.

Again, common sense should prevail. The dentist's primary aim is not to cure a patient's dental phobia but to reduce the anxiety sufficiently to permit reasonable access and allow the treatment to proceed. Patients who want to be cured of their phobias should go to a behavior therapist and participate in a comprehensive treatment program that takes into account their life-styles, social relationships, and personal history in addition to the presenting phobic symptoms. Dental patients seeking to have their anxiety reduced as a specific means of tolerating dental procedures cannot expect to receive such extensive treatment, as it would be beyond the resources of most dental practices. However, both patient and dentist would benefit from an apprehensive patient having access to some of the techniques known to be effective in reducing anxiety.

Social Psychology and Patient Management

The evidence and arguments presented strongly suggest that most of the procedures employed in patient management are affected by the quality of the relationship between the dentist and the patient. Here again, common sense must prevail. It is clearly impractical for a dentist to form a close personal relationship with all of the hundreds of patients in the practice. Some patients are less likeable than others, some do not wish to have a personal connection with their dentist, many do not attend frequently enough to allow a relationship to develop. However, as has been indicated previously, most dentists could do a great deal more to foster a close relationship with those patients receptive to such an idea. Not only would this facilitate patient management, it would also increase the job satisfaction of the dentist.

Research in the Psychology of Dentistry: Problems

There is no dearth of research investigating the psychology of dentistry. What is lacking is high quality research. Many of the articles tend to be polemical rather than empiric in that they advocate a particular course of action without providing supporting evidence for the recommendations. Other reports tend to be case studies of a few individuals, on the basis of which the authors then tend to overgeneralize their results. And there is a whole body of literature that has been influenced by Freudian theory, which is of more interest to psychoanalysts than to dentists.

There are several reasons for the relative lack of significant research. Most dentists are not trained in the methods and theory of social science and are therefore not in a very good position to conceptualize and implement psychologic studies. Another major problem, not unique to this field, is the universally acknowledged difficulty of conducting interdisciplinary research. Psychologists who wish to inquire into the dentist-patient relationship must first establish a connection with a dentist and persuade that person to cooperate in research. Next, psychologists must make themselves familiar with the practices, issues and problems of dentistry, translate these into the language of social science, and then explain this transformation to the dentist. Non-psychologists often want psychologists to ask questions that cannot be directly posed for various reasons, and become impatient with the circuitous logic and cumbersome statistical analyses that characterize much social science research. Unfortunately, there are many topics and questions that cannot be addressed directly without serious methodologic consequences, something that non-psychologists often find frustrating and difficult to accept.

Another reason for the paucity of good research is the difficulty in gaining access to subjects. The dental appointment is already crammed to the limit with other procedures, not allowing much time or scope for collecting psychologic data. The pre-appointment time may not be an entirely suitable occasion for research because the subjects may be anxious. In the post-appointment phase subjects may be suffering pain, or be sedated. More generally, subjects must consent to be interviewed or studied, both on ethical and practical grounds. Some people may regard psychologic research as an intrusion into their privacy, particularly when it is taking place during a period when they are already under stress. For the same reason many dentists may not be willing to allow social scientists access to their patients, or conduct the research themselves for fear of antagonizing their patients.

The solution to the problem of research training, interdisciplinary cooperation, and subject access lies in the hands of the professional dental associations. These organizations represent the collective views and interests of their members, and are in a position to influence training, arrange and facilitate interdisciplinary projects, and encourage individual members to throw open the doors of their surgeries to social science research. These bodies can also disseminate the results of such research to their members and thereby diffuse improved methods into the health care delivery system.

Research in the Psychology of Dentistry: Topics and Strategies

It would be inappropriate and indeed impossible to itemize a list of topics that should receive detailed investigation. The reality of research is that a particular topic is chosen because a particular investigator has a special interest in it *and* because there is an opportunity to follow up the idea. A much more practical approach is to distinguish between various research strategies and indicate their relative usefulness, thereby setting up general guidelines for studies investigating the dentist-patient relationship.

The Shotgun Survey

The least useful kind of research project is the shotgun survey in which the investigator asks many unrelated questions and then tries to make sense of the data afterwards. Such studies can be contrasted with the survey that has a specific rationale on which it is based. For instance, an investigator may be interested in the incidence of dental phobia. In this case, the research effort would go into developing suitable measures of dental aversion. Next, after giving due consideration to sampling requirements, a large number of patients would be given the survey, the contents of which would all converge on the topic under scrutiny—dental apprehension. Any other items in the questionnaire would be included strictly only if they were germane to the central purpose of the research program. If such a strategy is followed, all the data can be easily interpreted because they form part of a coherent pattern.

Case Studies

There are a great many reports of case studies in the literature. The term "case study" here refers to a subjective description of a procedure, outcome, or incident, the observations based on one, two, or at most a handful of subjects. Such reports can be useful in generating hypotheses but tend to be misleading if the author or the reader generalize the results to a class of patients. Nothing divides the physical from the social sciences more than the issue of sampling. Physical scientists often conduct useful research with very small samples because there may be fewer individual differences in their domain. For instance, if a particular anesthetic can be shown to work with one patient, the chances are it will probably work with most patients. Not so in the social sciences. There are large individual differences in the way that people respond psychologically, depending on who they are and what is presented to them. Consequently, samples have to be large and representative, the subjects being either randomly allocated to experimental conditions or systematically selected for certain predetermined characteristics. Most case studies pay no heed to sampling requirements and their results therefore cannot be generalized beyond the particular patients who served in the studies, or patients exactly like them. In that sense case studies lack utility because their insights may not apply in other contexts.

Atheoretical Practical Questions

There are many studies in the literature that address themselves to a specific, practical issue. Some examples include the following: Should dentists wear a uniform or informal clothing? What is the optimal length of an appointment? Does the surgery arouse more anxiety than the waiting room? Should mothers be present or absent during their child's treatment? Is one form of behavior therapy more effective than another? The questions could go on, and many dentists reading this section can undoubtedly extend the list considerably from their own curiosity about patient behavior. Indeed, practicing dentists are the most likely sources of ideas for studies of this nature.

There is nothing intrinsically wrong with such pragmatic research, and it is certainly vastly preferable to seek an empiric answer to a question rather than speculate about it in the armchair. The problem is that even if an answer to a particular question has been obtained in this way, the explanation for the phenomenon is still lacking. Let us assume that patients in a surgery with piped music were found to be less anxious than patients in a surgery that did not have this facility. That would be an interesting finding but would not tell us why and how music decreased anxiety. To answer that question, it would be necessary to carry out an experiment that was derived from some general theory of behavior.

Theory-Based Research

The most useful studies are those that have a rationale based on a general theory because such studies provide an account or explanation of the phenomenon. For example, cognitive balance theory (Heider, 1958) states that there is a strain towards consistency in our cognitive systems. Applied to attitude change, this theorem implies that high credible communicators will be more effective in changing opinions than low credible ones because high credible persons are more difficult to disparage than low credible sources. It is cognitively inconsistent to regard someone as highly credible and then disparage what they advocate; hence under these circumstances the dissonance set up by the persuasive communication is reduced by agreeing with the communicator. These theoretic ideas have all kinds of implications for dental health education. For instance, the theory suggests the hypothesis that dentists who are highly regarded by their patients will be more effective health educators than less trusted dentists, because the former are more difficult to disparage and ignore than the latter. However, this conclusion cannot be drawn without actually conducting the experiment, because there may be elements in dental health communications that cancel out or counteract the forces operating in other areas of social influence.

The proponents of theory-based research frequently have to contend with the ill-informed criticism that they are proving the obvious. It is certainly true that such research provides a rationale for the outcome before the results have been obtained but this predictive aspect is precisely what makes the procedure so elegant and powerful. However, usually the rationale offered is only one of several competing plausible explanations and until the experiments have been conducted, the various explanations have only the status of hypotheses. Systematic research consists of ruling out all plausible alternate hypotheses until the most likely explanation is revealed. The true scientist is the complete skeptic, rejecting that any phenomenon is obvious or self-evident until this has been confirmed through rigorous study.

Dentists are unlikely to be familiar with the more arcane content of the social sciences and therefore cannot be expected to initiate sophisticated, theory-based research projects. This implies that theoretically inspired, programmatic research depends on multidisciplinary cooperation, and explains why such investigations are not much in evidence in the literature.

Conclusion

This book was written for the dental researcher and practitioner. The aim has been to bring to the fore what social science has to say about dental practice. The main issues, controversies, findings, and recommendations have been presented and critically reviewed. The book has also tried to lay to rest some of the myths current about the dentist-patient relationship. There has been an attempt to provide general guidelines for the form as distinct from the content of useful research.

Dentists are highly trained, highly skilled professionals who provide a most useful service to society. The nature of their work results in stress for themselves and for their patients. This stress can be relieved, although not eliminated with methods, techniques, and ideas that originate in the social sciences. Social scientists for their part would regard the dental surgery as an ideal setting to study a host of problems that they are concerned with, such as anxiety reduction, stereotyping, or attitude change. Only good can come out of greater cooperation in the future between dentists and social scientists. However, such cooperation is only feasible if these diverse professionals are aware of each other's concerns and problems. A major aim of this book has been an attempt to bridge this gap.

References

Ackerman, C.A., & Endler, N.S. (1985). The interaction model of anxiety and dental treatment. *Journal of Research in Personality, 19*, 78–88.

Adelson, R., & Goldfried, M.R. (1970). Modeling and the fearful child patient. *Journal of Dentistry for Children, 37*, 34–47.

Agras, S., Sylvester, D., & Oliveau, D. (1969). The epidemiology of common fears and phobia. *Comprehensive Psychiatry, 10*, 151–156.

Ajzen, I., & Fishbein, M. (1980). *Understanding attitudes and predicting social behavior.* Englewood Cliffs, N.J.: Prentice-Hall.

Allport, G.W. (1954). The historical background of modern social psychology. In G. Lindzey (Ed.), *Handbook of social psychology. Volume 1.* Cambridge, Mass.: Addison-Wesley.

Allport, G.W. (1958). *The nature of prejudice.* Garden City, N.Y.: Doubleday Anchor.

Aronson, E. (1976). *The social animal. Second edition.* San Francisco: W.H. Freeman.

Ayer, W.A., & Gale, E.N. (1970). Psychology and thumbsucking. Journal of the American Dental Association, *80*, 1335–1337.

Bailey, C., Dey, F., Reynolds, K., Rutter, G., Teoh, T., & Peck, C. (1981). What are the variables related to dental compliance? *Australian Dental Journal, 26*, 46–48.

Bailey, P.M., Talbot, A., & Taylor, P.P. (1973). A comparison of maternal anxiety levels with anxiety levels manifested in the child dental patient. *Journal of Dentistry for Children, 40*, 277–284.

Bandura, A. (1977). *Social learning theory.* Englewood Cliffs, N.J.: Prentice-Hall.

Bandura, A. (1983). Self-efficacy determinants of anticipated fears and calamities. *Journal of Personality and Social Psychology, 45*, 464–469.

Bandura, A., Blanchard, E.B., & Ritter, B. (1969). Relative efficacy of desensitization and modeling approaches for inducing behavioral, affective and attitudinal changes. *Journal of Personality and Social Psychology, 13*, 173–199.

Bandura, A., Grusec, J.E., & Menlove, F.L. (1967). Vicarious extinction of avoidance behavior. *Journal of Personality and Social Psychology, 5*, 16–23.

Bandura, A., Reese, L., & Adams, N.E. (1982). Microanalysis of action and fear arousal as a function of differential levels of perceived self-efficacy. *Journal of Personality and Social Psychology, 43*, 5–21.

Barker, R.G. (1968). *Ecological psychology: Concepts and methods for studying the environment of human behavior.* Stanford, Calif.: Stanford University Press.

Barker, R.G. (1979). Settings of a professional lifetime. *Journal of Personality and Social Psychology, 37*, 2137–2157.

Barnard, P.D. (1976). Dental conditions in high school students, Sydney, 1972. *Australian Dental Journal, 21*, 513–516.

Basmajian, J.V. (Ed.). (1979). *Biofeedback: Principles and practice for clinicians.* Baltimore: Williams and Wilkins.

Bates, M.S. (1987). Ethnicity and pain: A biocultural model. *Social Science and Medicine, 24*, 47–50.

Bayer, T.L. (1985). Weaving a tangled web: The psychology of deception and self deception in psychogenic pain. *Social Science and Medicine, 20*, 517–527.

Beck, F.M. (1977). Placebos in dentistry: Their profound potential effects. *Journal of the American Dental Association, 95*, 1122–1126.

Beck, F.M., Kaul, T.J., & Weaver II, J.M. (1979). Recognition and management of the depressed dental patient. *Journal of the American Dental Association, 99*, 967–971.

Beck, F.M., & Weaver II, J.M. (1981). Blood pressure and heart rate responses to anticipated high-stress dental treatment. *Journal of Dental Research, 60*, 26–29.

Beecher, H.K. (1956). Relationship of significance of wound to pain experienced. *The Journal of the American Medical Association, 161*, 1609–1613.

Beecher, H.K. (1972). The placebo effect as a non-specific force surrounding disease and the treatment of disease. In R. Janzen, W.D. Keidel, A. Herz, C. Steichele, J.P. Payne, & R.A.P. Burt (Eds.), *Pain: Basic principles—pharmacology—therapy.* Stuttgart: Georg Thieme.

Beecroft, R.S. (1966). *Classical conditioning.* Goleta, Calif.: Psychonomic Press.

Bem, S.L. (1974). The measurement of psychological androgyny. *Journal of Consulting and Clinical Psychology, 42*, 155–162.

Berggren, U., & Carlsson, S.G. (1984). A psychophysiological therapy for dental fear. *Behavior Research and Therapy, 22*, 487–492.

Bernstein, D.A., Kleinknecht, R.A., & Alexander, L.B. (1979). Antecedents of dental fear. *Journal of Public Health Dentistry, 39*, 113–124.

Birbaumer, N., Elbert, T., Rockstroh, B., & Lutzenberger, W. (1981). Biofeedback of event-related slow potentials of the brain. *International Journal of Psychology, 16*, 389–415.

Biro, P.A., & Hewson, N.D. (1976). A survey of patients' attitudes to their dentist. *Australian Dental Journal, 21*, 388–394.

Bishop, T.G., Flett, R.D., and Beck, D.J. (1975). A survey of dental health knowledge and attitudes in Owaka, a rural community in South Otago. *New Zealand Dental Journal, 71*, 185–190.

Blaikie, D.C. (1979). Cultural barriers to preventive dentistry. *Australian Dental Journal, 24*, 398–401.

Blandford, D.H., & Dane, J.K. (1981). Problems in dental practice: A pilot study for continuing education. *Journal of the American Dental Association, 103*, 869–874.

Bochner, S. (1980). Unobtrusive methods in cross-cultural experimentation. In H.C. Triandis & J.W. Berry (Eds.), *Handbook of cross-cultural psychology: Methodology. Volume 2.* Boston: Allyn and Bacon.

Bochner, S., & Insko, C.A. (1966). Communicator discrepancy, source credibility, and opinion change. *Journal of Personality and Social Psychology, 4*, 614–621.

Bochner, S., Ivanoff, P., & Watson, J. (1974). Organisation development in the A.B.C. *Personnel Practice Bulletin, 30*, 219–233.

Borkovec, T.D., & Sides, J.K. (1979). Critical procedural variables related to the physiological effects of progressive relaxation: A review. *Behaviour Research and Therapy, 17*, 119–125.

Boulougouris, J.C., & Marks, I.M. (1969). Implosion (flooding)—a new treatment for phobias. *British Medical Journal, 2*, 721–723.

Braginsky, D.D., & Braginsky, B.M. (1976). The myth of schizophrenia. In P.A. Magaro (Ed.), *The construction of madness: Emerging conceptions and interventions into the psychotic process.* Oxford: Pergamon.

Brown, J.P., & Smith, I.T. (1979). Childhood fear and anxiety states in relation to dental treatment. *Australian Dental Journal, 24*, 256–259.

Buglass, D., Clarke, J., Henderson, A.S., Kreitman, N., & Presley, A.S. (1977). A study of agoraphobic housewives. *Psychological Medicine, 7*, 73–86.

Bureau of Economic Research and Statistics. (1975). Mortality of dentists, 1968 to 1972. *Journal of the American Dental Association, 90*, 195–198.

Campbell, D.T. (1967). Stereotypes and the perception of group differences. *American Psychologist, 22*, 817–829.

Carlsson, S.G., Linde, A., & Ohman, A. (1980). Reduction of tension in fearful dental patients. *Journal of the American Dental Association, 101*, 638–641.

Carr, L.M. (1982). Dental health of children in Australia 1977–1980. *Australian Dental Journal, 27*, 169–175.

Castenada, A., McCandless, B.R., & Palmero, D.S. (1956). The children's form of the Manifest Anxiety Scale. *Child Development, 27*, 317–326.

Cattell, R.B. (1965). *The scientific analysis of personality.* Baltimore: Penguin.

Cerny, R. (1981). Thumb and finger sucking. *Australian Dental Journal, 26*, 167–171.

Chambers, D.W. (1977). Patient susceptibility limits to the effectiveness of preventive oral health education. *Journal of the American Dental Association, 95*, 1159–1163.

Chen, M., & Rubinson, L. (1982). Preventive dental behavior in families: A national survey. *Journal of the American Dental Association, 105*, 43–46.

Christen, A.G., Park, P.R., Graves, R.C., Young, J.M., & Rahe, A.J. (1979). United States Air Force survey of dental needs, 1977: Methodology and summary of findings. *Journal of the American Dental Association, 98*, 726–730.

Cipes, M.H., & Miraglia, M. (1985). Pedodontists' attitudes toward parental presence during children's dental visits. *Journal of Dentistry for Children, 52*, 341–343.

Cipes, M.H., Miraglia, M., & Gaulin-Kremer, E. (1986). Monitoring and reinforcement to eliminate thumbsucking. *Journal of Dentistry for Children, 53*, 48–52.

Clark, A.W., & Powell, R.J. (1984). Changing drivers' attitudes through peer group decision. *Human Relations, 37*, 155–162.

Clarke, J.C., & Jackson, A.J. (1983). *Hypnosis and behavior therapy: The treatment of anxiety and phobias.* New York: Springer.

Cohen, S.D. (1973). Children's attitudes toward dentists' attire. *Journal of Dentistry for Children, 40*, 285–287.

Collett, H.A. (1969). Influence of dentist-patient relationship on attitudes and adjustment to dental treatment. *Journal of the American Dental Association, 79*, 879–884.

Congalton, A.A. (1969). *Status and prestige in Australia.* Melbourne: Cheshire.

Cooper, C.L., Mallinger, M., & Kahn, R.L. (1980). Dentistry: What causes it to be a stressful occupation? *International Review of Applied Psychology, 29*, 307–319.

Cooper, C.L., Watts, J., & Kelly, M. (1987). Job satisfaction, mental health, and job stressors among general dental practitioners in the UK. *British Dental Journal, 162*, 77–81.

Corah, N.L. (1969). Development of a dental anxiety scale. *Journal of Dental Research, 48*, 596.

Corah, N.L. (1973). Effect of perceived control on stress reduction in pedodontic patients. *Journal of Dental Research, 52*, 1261–1264.

Corah, N.L., Bissell, G.D., & Illig, S.J. (1978). Effect of perceived control on stress reduction in adult dental patients. *Journal of Dental Research, 57*, 74–76.

Corah, N.L., Gale, E.N., & Illig, S.J. (1978). Assessment of a dental anxiety scale. *Journal of the American Dental Association, 97*, 816–819.

Corah, N.L., Gale, E.N., & Illig, S.J. (1979a). The use of relaxation and distraction to reduce psychological stress during dental procedures. *Journal of the American Dental Association, 98*, 390–394.

Corah, N.L., Gale, E.N., & Illig, S.J. (1979b). Psychological stress reduction during dental procedures. *Journal of Dental Research, 58*, 1347–1351.

Corah, N.L., O'Shea, R.M., & Ayer, W.A. (1985). Dentists' management of patients' fear and anxiety. *Journal of the American Dental Association, 110*, 734–736.

Cosgrove, D. (1976). Sedation in dentistry. *Australian Dental Journal, 21*, 128–130.

Crano, W.D., & Brewer, M.B. (1973). *Principles of research in social psychology*. New York: McGraw-Hill.

Crowne, D.P., & Marlowe, D. (1964). *The approval motive*. New York: Wiley.

Cutright, D.E., Carpenter, W.A., Tsaknis, P.G., & Lyon, T.C. (1977). Survey of blood pressures of 856 dentists. *Journal of the American Dental Association, 94*, 918–919.

Darley, J.M., & Latane, B. (1968). Bystander intervention in emergencies: Diffusion of responsibility. *Journal of Personality and Social Psychology, 8*, 377–383.

De la Rosa, M. (1978). Dental caries and socioeconomic status in Mexican children. *Journal of Dental Research, 57*, 453–457.

DePaulo, B.M., & Coleman, L.M. (1986). Talking to children, foreigners, and retarded adults. *Journal of Personality and Social Psychology, 51*, 945–959.

Deneen, L.J., Heid, D.W., & Smith, A.A. (1973). Effective interpersonal and management skills in dentistry. *Journal of the American Dental Association, 87*, 878–880.

Denney, D.R. (1974). Active, passive, and vicarious desensitization. *Journal of Counseling Psychology, 21*, 369–375.

Dennison, D., Lucye, H., & Suomi, J.D. (1974). Effects of dental health instruction on university students. *Journal of the American Dental Association, 89*, 1313–1317.

Donaldson, C., Forbes, J.F., Smalls, M., Boddy, F.A., Stephen, K.W., & McCall, D. (1986). Preventive dentistry in a health centre: Effectiveness and cost. *Social Science and Medicine, 23*, 861–868.

Eiser, J.R. (1982). Addiction as attribution: Cognitive processes in giving up smoking. In J.R. Eiser (Ed.), *Social psychology and behavioral medicine*. Chichester: Wiley.

Eiser, J.R. (1986). *Social Psychology: Attitudes, cognitions and social behaviour*. Cambridge: Cambridge University Press.

Eli, I. (1984). Professional socialization in dentistry: A longitudinal analysis of changes in students' expected professional rewards. *Social Science and Medicine, 18*, 297–302.

Endler, N.S., & Hunt, J. McV. (1968). S-R inventories of hostility and comparisons of the proportions of variance from persons, responses, and situations for hostility and anxiousness. *Journal of Personality and Social Psychology, 9*, 309–315.

Endler, N.S., & Magnusson, D. (1976). *Interactional psychology and personality*. New York: Wiley.

Erwin, E. (1980). Psychoanalytic therapy: The Eysenck argument. *American Psychologist, 35*, 435–443.

Estabrook, B., Zapka, J., & Lubin, H. (1980). Consumer perceptions of dental care in the health services program of an educational institution. *Journal of the American Dental Association, 100*, 540–543.

Ettinger, R.L., Beck, J.D., & Glenn, R.E. (1979). Eliminating office architectural barriers to dental care of the elderly and handicapped. *Journal of the American Dental Association, 98*, 398–401.

Evans, R.I. (1982). Training social psychologists in behavioral medicine research. In J.R. Eiser (Ed.), *Social psychology and behavioral medicine*. Chichester: Wiley.

Eysenck, H.J. (1966). *The effects of psychotherapy*. New York: International Science Press.

Fadden, L.E. (1953). What the child thinks of dental practice. *New York State Dental Journal, 19*, 124–132.

Fanning, E.A., & Leppard, P.I. (1973). A survey of university students in South Australia. Part III. Attitudes to dental treatment. *Australian Dental Journal, 18*, 20–22.

Ferber, I., & Bedrick, A.E. (1979). Dental survey of 620 Soviet immigrants. *Journal of the American Dental Association, 98*, 379–383.

Festinger, L. (1954). A theory of social comparison processes. *Human Relations, 7*, 117–140.

Festinger, L. (1957). *A theory of cognitive dissonance*. Evanston, Ill.: Row, Peterson.

Festinger, L., & Carlsmith, J.M. (1959). Cognitive consequences of forced compliance. *Journal of Abnormal and Social Psychology, 58*, 203–210.

Fields, H., & Pinkham, J. (1976). Videotape modeling of the child dental patient. *Journal of Dental Research, 55*, 958–963.

Finer, B. (1972). The use of hypnosis in the clinical management of pain. In R. Janzen, W.D. Keidel, A. Herz, C. Steichele, J.P. Payne, & R.A.P. Burt (Eds.), *Pain: Basic principles—pharmacology—therapy*. Stuttgart: Georg Thieme.

Finnie, W.C. (1973). Field experiments in litter control. *Environment and Behavior, 5*, 123–144.

Fishbein, M. (1967). Attitude and prediction of behavior. In M. Fishbein (Ed.), *Readings in attitude theory and measurement*. New York: Wiley.

Fishbein, M. (1982). Social psychological analysis of smoking behavior. In J.R. Eiser (Ed.), *Social psychology and behavioral medicine*. Chichester: Wiley.

Frazier, P.J., Jenny, J., & Bagramian, R.A. (1974). Parents' descriptions of barriers faced and strategies used to obtain dental care. *Journal of Public Health Dentistry, 34*, 22–38.

Fredrikson, M., & Ohman, A. (1979). Cardiovascular and electrodermal responses conditioned to fear-relevant stimuli. *Psychophysiology, 16*, 1–7.

Freeman, R.E. (1985). Dental students as operators: Emotional reactions. *Medical Education, 19*, 27–33.

Friend, M.R. (1953). Everyday psychiatric problems of dentistry. *New York Journal of Dentistry, 23*, 252–257.

Fuller, N.P., Menke, R.A., & Meyers, W.J. (1979). Perception of pain to three different intraoral penetrations of needles. *Journal of the American Dental Association, 99*, 822–824.

Furnham, A. (1983). Social skills and dentistry. *British Dental Journal, 154*, 404–408.

Furnham, A., & Bochner, S. (1986). *Culture shock: Psychological reactions to unfamiliar environments.* London: Methuen.

Gaffney, T.J., Foenander, G., Reade, P.C., & Burrows, G.D. (1981). The personalities of dentists as a factor in the use of nitrous oxide relative analgesia. *Australian Dental Journal, 26*, 387–389.

Gale, E.N. (1972). Fears of the dental situation. *Journal of Dental Research, 51*, 964–966.

Garcia, J.A., & Juarez, R.Z. (1978). Utilization of dental health services by Chicanos and Anglos. *Journal of Health and Social Behavior, 19*, 428–436.

Garfield, S.L. (1981). Psychotherapy: A 40-year appraisal. *American Psychologist, 36*, 174–183.

Gatchel, R.J. (1980). Effectiveness of two procedures for reducing dental fear: Group-administered desensitization and group education and discussion. *Journal of the American Dental Association, 101*, 634–637.

Geller, E.S., Witmer, J.F., & Tuso, M.A. (1977). Environmental interventions for litter control. *Journal of Applied Psychology, 62*, 344–351.

George, J.M., & Scott, D.S. (1982). The effects of psychological factors on recovery from surgery. *Journal of the American Dental Association, 105*, 251–258.

Gerschman, J., Burrows, G., & Reade, P. (1978). Hypnotherapy in the treatment of oro-facial pain. *Australian Dental Journal, 23*, 492–496.

Gessel, A.H. (1975). Electromyographic biofeedback and tricyclic antidepressants in myofascial pain-dysfunction syndrome: Psychological predictors of outcome. *Journal of the American Dental Association, 91*, 1048–1052.

Gibb, C.A. (1954). Leadership. In G. Lindzey (Ed.), *Handbook of social psychology. Volume 2.* Cambridge, Mass.: Addison-Wesley.

Gibson, E.J., & Walk, R.D. (1960). The "visual cliff". *Scientific American, 202* (4), 64–71.

Gobetti, J.P. (1981). The psychological aspects of dental therapy: A diagnostic problem. *Journal of the American Dental Association, 102*, 662–663.

Gochman, D.S. (1972). The organizing role of motivation in health beliefs and intentions. *Journal of Health and Social Behavior, 13*, 285–293.

Goldfried, M.R., & Trier, C.S. (1974). Effectiveness of relaxation as an active coping skill. *Journal of Abnormal Psychology, 83*, 348–355.

Goodenough, F.L., & Tyler, L.E. (1959). *Developmental psychology: An introduction to the study of human behavior. Third Edition.* New York: Appleton-Century-Crofts.

Goodman, P., Greene, C.S., & Laskin, D.M. (1976). Response of patients with myofascial pain-dysfunction syndrome to mock equilibration. *Journal of the American Dental Association, 92*, 755–758.

Graham, G. (1974). Hypnoanalysis in dental practice. *American Journal of Clinical Hypnosis, 16*, 178–187.

Grainger, J.K. (1972). Perception: Its meaning, significance and control in dental procedures. Part III: Clinical aspects. *Australian Dental Journal, 17*, 204–208.

Greene, B.F., & Neistat, M.D. (1983). Behavior analysis in consumer affairs: Encouraging dental professionals to provide consumers with shielding from unnecessary X-ray exposure. *Journal of Applied Behavior Analysis, 16*, 13–27.

Greene, C.S., & Laskin, D.M. (1974). Long-term evaluation of conservative treatment for myofascial pain-dysfunction syndrome. *Journal of the American Dental Association, 89*, 1365–1368.

Grembowski, D., & Conrad, D.A. (1986). Coinsurance effects on dental prices. *Social

Science and Medicine, 23, 1131–1138.

Guilford, J.P. (1967). Response biases and response sets. In M. Fishbein (Ed.), *Readings in attitude theory and measurement.* New York: Wiley.

Gurling, F.G., Fanning, E.A., & Leppard, P.I. (1980). Handicapped children: Behavioural and co-ordination characteristics affecting the delivery of dental care. *Australian Dental Journal, 25*, 201–204.

Guthrie, E.R. (1952). *The psychology of learning. Revised edition.* New York: Harper.

Guthrie, G.M. (1975). A behavioral analysis of culture learning. In R.W. Brislin, S. Bochner, & W.J. Lonner (Eds.), *Cross-cultural perspectives on learning.* New York: Wiley.

Hall, E.T. (1959). *The silent language.* Garden City, N.Y.: Doubleday.

Hall, E.T. (1966). *The hidden dimension.* Garden City, N.Y.: Doubleday.

Haney, C., Banks, W.C., & Zimbardo, P.G. (1973). Interpersonal dynamics in a simulated prison. *International Journal of Criminology and Penology, 1*, 69–97.

Harris, B. (1979). Whatever happened to Little Albert? *American Psychologist, 34*, 151–160.

Heider, F. (1958). *The psychology of interpersonal relations.* New York: Wiley.

Herbertt, R.M., & Innes, J.M. (1979). Familiarization and preparatory information in the reduction of anxiety in child dental patients. *Journal of Dentistry for Children, 46*, 47–51.

Hilgard, E.R. (1973). A neodissociation interpretation of pain reduction in hypnosis. *Pychological Review, 80*, 396–411.

Hill, F.J., & O'Mullane, D.M. (1976). A preventive program for the dental management of frightened children. *Journal of Dentistry for Children, 43*, 30–34.

Hodgson, R., & Rachman, S. (1974). II. Desynchrony in measures of fear. *Behaviour Research and Therapy, 12*, 319–326.

Hoogstraten, J., de Haan, W., & Horst, G.T. (1985). Stimulating the demand for dental care: An application of Ajzen and Fishbein's theory of reasoned action. *European Journal of Social Psychology, 15*, 401–414.

Hornsby, J.L., Deneen, L.J., & Heid, D.W. (1975). Interpersonal communication skills development: A model for dentistry. *Journal of Dental Education, 39*, 728–732.

Horowitz, E.L. (1965). Development of attitude toward Negroes. In H. Proshansky & B. Seidenberg (Eds.), *Basic studies in social psychology.* New York: Holt, Rinehart and Winston.

Hovland, C.I., Janis, I.L., & Kelley, H.H. (1963). *Communication and persuasion: Psychological studies of opinion change.* New Haven: Yale University Press.

Hull, C.L. (1951). *Essentials of behavior.* New Haven: Yale University Press.

Hutt, M.L., & Gibby, R.G. (1961). *The mentally retarded child: Development, education, and guidance.* Boston: Allyn and Bacon.

Indresano, A.T., & Rooney, T.P. (1981). Outpatient management of mentally handicapped patients undergoing dental procedures. *Journal of the American Dental Association, 102*, 328–330.

Ingersoll, B.D. (1982). *Behavioral aspects in dentistry.* New York: Appleton-Century-Crofts.

Insko, C.A. (1967). *Theories of attitude change.* New York: Appleton-Century-Crofts.

Jackson, E. (1975). Establishing rapport I. Verbal interaction. *Journal of Oral Medicine, 30*, 105–110.

Jenny, J., Frazier, P.J., Bagramian, R.A., & Proshek, J.M. (1973). Parents' satisfaction and dissatisfaction with their children's dentist. *Journal of Public Health Dentistry, 33*, 211–221.

Johnson, J.B., Pinkham, J.R., & Kerber, P.E. (1979). Stress reactions of various judging groups to the child dental patient. *Journal of Dental Research, 58*, 1664–1671.

Johnson, R., & Baldwin, D.C., Jr. (1968). Relationship of maternal anxiety to the behavior of young children undergoing dental extraction. *Journal of Dental Research, 47*, 801–805.

Johnson, R., & Baldwin, D.C., Jr. (1969). Maternal anxiety and child behavior. *Journal of Dentistry for Children, 36*, 87–92.

Jones, E.E. (1964). *Ingratiation: A social psychological analysis.* New York: Appleton-Century-Crofts.

Jones, E.E., & Nisbett, R.E. (1971). The actor and observer: Divergent perceptions of the causes of behavior. In E.E. Jones, D.E. Kanouse, H.H. Kelley, R.E. Nisbett, S. Valins, & B. Weiner (Eds.), *Attribution: Perceiving the causes of behavior.* Morristown, N.J.: General Learning Press.

Jorgenson, D.O., & Dukes, F.O. (1976). Deindividuation as a function of density and group membership. *Journal of Personality and Social Psychology, 34*, 24–29.

Katz, D., & Braly, K. (1933). Racial stereotypes of one hundred college students. *Journal of Abnormal and Social Psychology, 28*, 280–290.

Katz, D., & Braly, K. (1935). Racial prejudice and racial stereotypes. *Journal of Abnormal and Social Psychology, 30*, 175–193.

Katz, E. (1965). The two-step flow of communication: An up-to-date report on an hypothesis. In H. Proshansky & B. Seidenberg (Eds.), *Basic studies in social psychology.* New York: Holt, Rinehart and Winston.

Kazdin, A.E., & Wilcoxon, L.A. (1976). Systematic desensitization and nonspecific treatment effects: A methodological evaluation. *Psychological Bulletin, 83*, 729–758.

Kegeles, S.S. (1974). Why and how people use dental services. *International Dentistry Journal, 24*, 347–351.

Kent, G. (1983). Psychology in the dental curriculum. *British Dental Journal, 154*, 106–109.

Kent. G. (1984). Anxiety, pain and type of dental procedure. *Behaviour Research and Therapy, 22*, 465–469.

Kent, G. (1986). The typicality of therapeutic 'surprises'. *Behaviour Research and Therapy, 24*, 625–628.

Kent. G., & Gibbons, R. (1987). Self-efficacy and the control of anxious cognitions. *Journal of Behaviour Therapy and Experimental Psychiatry, 18*, 33–40.

Kerebel, L.M., Le Cabellec, M.T., Daculsi, G., & Kerebel, B. (1985). Report on caries reduction in French schoolchildren three years after the introduction of a preventive program. *Community Dentistry and Oral Epidemiology, 13*, 201–204.

Kerebel, L.M., Le Cabellec, M.T., Kerebel, B., & Daculsi, G. (1985). Effect of motivation on the oral health of French schoolchildren. *Journal of Dentistry for Children, 52*, 287–292.

Keys, J. (1978). Detecting and treating dental phobic children: Part I, detection. *Journal of Dentistry for Children, 45*, 296–300.

Keys, J., Field, M., & Korboot, P. (1978). Detecting and treating dental phobic children: Part II, treatment. *Journal of Dentistry for Children, 45*, 301–305.

Kimble, G.A. (1961). *Hilgard and Marquis' conditioning and learning. Second edition.* New York: Appleton-Century-Crofts.

King, W.H. & Tucker, K.M. (1973). Dental problems of alcoholic and nonalcoholic psychiatric patients. *Quarterly Journal of Studies on Alcohol, 34*, 1208–1211.

Kirsch, A.J. (1974). The psychiatric view of the mouth. *New York Journal of Dentistry, 44*, 117–119.

Kleinknecht, R.A., Mahoney, E.R., Alexander, L.D., & Dworkin, S.F. (1986). Correspondence between subjective report of temporomandibular disorder symptoms and clinical findings. *Journal of the American Dental Association, 113*, 257–261.

Kleinknecht, R.A., Klepac, R.K., & Alexander, L.D. (1973). Origins and characteristics of fear of dentistry. *Journal of the American Dental Association, 86*, 842–848.

Klepac, R.K., Dowling, J., Hauge, G., & McDonald, M. (1980). Reports of pain after dental treatment, electrical tooth pulp stimulation, and cutaneous shock. *Journal of the American Dental Association, 100*, 692–695.

Klineberg, O. (1966). *The human dimension in international relations.* New York: Holt, Rinehart and Winston.

Klinge, V. (1979). Facilitating oral hygiene in patients with chronic schizophrenia. *Journal of the American Dental Association, 99*, 644–645.

Klorman, R., Michael, R., Hilpert, P.L., & Sveen, O.B. (1979). A further assessment of predictors of the child's behavior in dental treatment. *Journal of Dental Research, 58*, 2338–2343.

Klorman, R., Ratner, J., Arata, C.L.G., King, J.B., Jr., & Sveen, O.B. (1978). Predicting the child's uncooperativeness in dental treatment from maternal trait, state, and dental anxiety. *Journal of Dentistry for Children, 45*, 62–67.

Koch, S. (1981). The nature and limits of psychological knowledge: Lessons of a century qua "science". *American Psychologist, 36*, 257–269.

Krauss, R.M., Freedman, J.L., & Whitcup, M. (1978). Field and laboratory studies of littering. *Journal of Experimental Social Psychology, 14*, 109–122.

Lamb, D.H., & Plant, R. (1972). Patient anxiety in the dentist's office. *Journal of Dental Research, 51*, 986–989.

Lambert, C. (1980). Psychological complications from the use of hypnosedatives in dental practice. *Australian Dental Journal, 25*, 81–83.

Lambert, W.E., Libman, E., & Poser, E.G. (1960). The effect of increased salience of a membership group on pain tolerance. *Journal of Personality, 28*, 350–357.

Laskin, D.M., & Greene, C.S. (1972). Influence of the doctor-patient relationship on placebo therapy for patients with myofascial pain-dysfunction (MPD) syndrome. *Journal of the American Dental Association, 85*, 892–894.

Lautch, H. (1971). Dental phobia. *British Journal of Psychiatry, 119*, 151–158.

Lawson, W.R., Jr. (1980). Children and dental care: Charges and probability of a visit by individual characteristics. *Journal of the American Dental Association, 101*, 32–37.

Lazarus, A.A. (1971). *Behavior therapy and beyond.* New York: McGraw-Hill.

Lenchner, V. (1966). The effect of appointment length on behavior of the pedodontic patient and his attitude toward dentistry. *Journal of Dentistry for Children, 33*, 61–74.

Leventhal, H., Brown, D., Shacham, S., & Engquist, G. (1979). Effects of preparatory information about sensations, threat of pain, and attention on cold pressor distress. *Journal of Personality and Social Psychology, 37*, 688–714.

Lewin, K. (1947) Group decision and social change. In T.M. Newcomb & E.L. Hartley (Eds.), *Readings in social psychology.* New York: Holt, Rinehart and Winston.

Liddell, A., & May, B. (1984). Some characteristics of regular and irregular attenders for dental check-ups. *British Journal of Clinical Psychology, 23*, 19–26.

Lin, N. (1976). *Foundations of social research.* New York: McGraw-Hill.

Lindsay, S.J.E. (1984). The fear of dental treatment: A critical and theoretical analysis. In S. Rachman (Ed.), *Contributions to medical psychology. Volume 3.* Oxford: Pergamon.

Lindsay, S.J.E., & Woolgrove, J.C. (1982). Fear and pain in dentistry. *Bulletin of the British Psychological Society, 35,* 225–228.

Linn, E.L. (1974). What dental patients don't know about preventive care. *Journal of Public Health Dentistry, 34,* 39–41.

Linn, E.L. (1976). Teenagers' attitudes, knowledge, and behaviors related to oral health. *Journal of the American Dental Association, 92,* 946–951.

Liska, A.E. (1974). Emergent issues in the attitude-behavior consistency controversy. *American Sociological Review, 39,* 261–272.

Lovibond, S.H., Mithiran, & Adams, W.G. (1979). The effects of three experimental prison environments on the behaviour of non-convict volunteer subjects. *Australian Psychologist, 14,* 273–285.

Lundberg, O. (1986). Class and health: Comparing Britain and Sweden. *Social Science and Medicine, 23,* 511–517.

Macgregor, I.D.M., & Rugg-Gunn, A.J. (1986). Effect of filming on toothbrushing performance in uninstructed adults in north-east England. *Community Dentistry and Oral Epidemiology, 14,* 320–322.

Machen, J.B., & Johnson, R. (1974). Desensitization, model learning, and the dental behavior of children. *Journal of Dental Research, 53,* 83–87.

MacIntyre, S. (1986). The patterning of health by social position in contemporary Britain: Directions for sociological research. *Social Science and Medicine, 23,* 393–415.

Maguire, P. (1981). Doctor-patient skills. In M. Argyle (Ed.), *Social skills and health.* London: Methuen.

Makkes, P.C., Schuurs, A.H.B., van Velzen, S.K.T., Duivenvoorden, H.J., & Verhage, F. (1986). Clinical measurement of dental anxiety. *Community Dentistry and Oral Epidemiology, 14,* 184.

Mann, L. (1974). On being a sore loser: How fans react to their team's failure. *Australian Journal of Psychology, 26,* 37–47.

Marano, P.D. (1977). Psychological benefits of oral surgery: Report of case. *Journal of the American Dental Association, 94,* 705–707.

Marbach, J.J., & Dworkin, S.F. (1975). Chronic MPD, group therapy, and psychodynamics. *Journal of the American Dental Association, 90,* 827–833.

Marks, I.M. (1969). *Fears and phobias.* London: Heinemann.

Martin, R.T. (1965). *An exploratory investigation of the dentist/patient relation.* Sydney: The Dental Health Education and Research Foundation of the University of Sydney.

Martin, R.T. (1970). *An investigation of the attitude and adjustment of practising dentists and dental students to their profession.* Sydney: The Dental Health Education and Research Foundation of the University of Sydney.

Mathews, A., & Rezin, V. (1977). Treatment of dental fears by imaginal flooding and rehearsal of coping behaviour. *Behaviour Research and Therapy, 15,* 321–328.

McCreary, C.P., & Gershen, J.A. (1978). Self and peer perception of male and female dental students. *Journal of Public Health Dentistry, 38,* 223–226.

McGlynn, F.D., McNeil, D.W., Gallagher, S.L., & Vrana, S. (1987). Factor structure, stability, and internal consistency of the dental fear survey. *Behavioral Assessment, 9,* 57–66.

Melamed, B.G. (1979). Behavioral approaches to fear in dental settings. In M. Hersen, R.M. Eisler, & P.M. Miller (Eds.), *Progress in behavior modification. Volume 7.* New York: Academic Press.

Melamed, B.G., Weinstein, D., Hawes, R., & Katin-Borland, M. (1975). Reduction of fear-related dental management problems with use of filmed modeling. *Journal of the American Dental Association, 90*, 822–826.

Meldman, M.J. (1972). The dental-phobia test. *Psychosomatics, 13*, 371–372.

Melzack, R., & Torgerson, W.S. (1971). On the language of pain. *Anesthesiology, 34*, 50–59.

Melzack, R., and Wall, P.D. (1984). *The challenge of pain*. Harmondsworth: Penguin.

Mercuri, L.G., Olson, R.E., & Laskin, D.M. (1979). The specificity of response to experimental stress in patients with myofascial pain dysfunction syndrome. *Journal of Dental Research, 58*, 1866–1871.

Messer, J.G. (1977). Stress in dental patients undergoing routine procedures. *Journal of Dental Research, 56*, 362–367.

Miller, H. (1974). Involving the dental patient, the new team member, in health awareness. *New York State Dental Journal, 40*, 280–282.

Mischel, W. (1968). *Personality and assessment*. New York: Wiley.

Moore, R., Miller, M.L., Weinstein, P., Dworkin, S.F., & Liou, H. (1986). Cultural perceptions of pain and pain coping among patients and dentists. *Community Dentistry and Oral Epidemiology, 14*, 327–333.

Mowrer, O.H. (1960a). *Learning theory and behavior*. New York: Wiley.

Mowrer, O.H. (1960b). *Learning theory and the symbolic processes*. New York: Wiley.

Neiburger, E.J. (1978). Child response to suggestion. *Journal of Dentistry for Children, 45*, 396–402.

Nevo, O., & Shapira, J. (1986). Use of humor in managing clinical anxiety. *Journal of Dentistry for Children, 53*, 97–100.

Nisbett, R.E., & Schachter, S. (1966). Cognitive manipulation of pain. *Journal of Experimental Social Psychology, 2*, 227–236.

Nunn, J.H., & Murray, J.J. (1987). The dental health of handicapped children in Newcastle and Northumberland. *British Dental Journal, 162*, 9–14.

O'Shea, R.M., Corah, N.L., & Ayer, W.A. (1983). Dentists' perceptions of the 'good' adult patient: An exploratory study. *Journal of the American Dental Association, 106*, 813–816.

O'Shea, R.M., Corah, N.L., & Ayer, W.A. (1984). Sources of dentists' stress. *Journal of the American Dental Association, 109*, 48–51.

Ohman, A. (1981). The role of experimental psychology in the scientific analysis of psychopathology. *International Journal of Psychology, 16*, 299–321.

Ohman, A., Eriksson, A., & Olofsson, C. (1975). One-trial learning and superior resistance to extinction of autonomic responses conditioned to potentially phobic stimuli. *Journal of Comparative and Physiological Psychology, 88*, 619–627.

Ohman, A., Fredrikson, M., Hugdahl, K., & Rimmo, P. (1976). The premise of equipotentiality in human classical conditioning: Conditioned electrodermal responses to potentially phobic stimuli. *Journal of Experimental Psychology: General, 105*, 313–337.

Orne, M.T. (1962). On the social psychology of the psychological experiment: With particular reference to demand characteristics and their implications. *American Psychologist, 17*, 776–783.

Orne, M.T. (1976). Mechanisms of hypnotic pain control. In J.J. Bonica & D.G. Albe-Fessard (Eds.), *Advances in pain research and therapy. Volume 1*. New York: Raven.

Ozar, D.T. (1985). Three models of professionalism and professional obligation in dentistry. *Journal of the American Dental Association, 110*, 173–177.

Packard, V. (1961). *The status seekers: An exploration of class behaviour in America*. Harmondsworth: Penguin Books.

Pavlov, I.P. (1927). *Conditioned reflexes*. London: Oxford University Press.

Pendleton, D.A., & Bochner, S. (1980). The communication of medical information in general practice consultations as a function of patients' social class. *Social Science and Medicine, 14A*, 669–673.

Pillard, R.C., & Fisher, S. (1970). Aspects of anxiety in dental clinic patients. *Journal of the American Dental Association, 80*, 1331–1334.

Pomp, A.M. (1974). Psychotherapy for the myofascial pain-dysfunction syndrome: A study of factors coinciding with symptom remission. *Journal of the American Dental Association, 89*, 629–632.

Quinn, I. (1977). New Jersey dentists' opinions on women as associates. *Journal of the American Dental Association, 94*, 717–718.

Rachman, S. (1971). *The effects of psychotherapy*. Oxford: Pergamon.

Rachman, S., & Hodgson, R.I. (1974). Synchrony and desynchrony in fear and avoidance. *Behaviour Research and Therapy, 12*, 311–318.

Raginsky, B.B. (1968). Some aspects of psychology applied to dentistry. *Journal of the Canadian Dental Association, 34*, 73–78.

Rankin, J.A., & Harris, M.B. (1984). Dental anxiety: The patient's point of view. *Journal of the American Dental Association, 109*, 43–47.

Rankin, J.A., & Harris, M.B. (1985). Patients' preferences for dentists' behaviors. *Journal of the American Dental Association, 110*, 323–327.

Reisenzein, R. (1983). The Schachter theory of emotion: Two decades later. *Psychological Bulletin, 94*, 239–264.

Richards, N.D., Willcocks, A.J., Bulman, J.S., & Slack, G.L. (1965). A survey of the dental health and attitudes towards dentistry in two communities. *British Dental Journal, 118*, 199–205.

Rimm, D.C., Janda, L.H., Lancaster, D.W., Nahl, M., & Dittmar, K. (1977). An exploratory investigation of the origin and maintenance of phobias. *Behaviour Research and Therapy, 15*, 231–238.

Ross, M., & Olson, J.M. (1982). Placebo effects in medical research and practice. In J.R. Eiser (Ed.), *Social psychology and behavioral medicine*. Chichester: Wiley.

Rouleau, J., Ladouceur, R., & Dufour, L. (1981). Pre-exposure to the first dental treatment. *Journal of Dental Research, 60*, 30–34.

Rubin, Z. (1973). *Liking and loving: An invitation to social psychology*. New York: Holt, Rinehart and Winston.

Runyon, H.L., & Cohen, L.A. (1979). The effects of systematic human relations training on freshman dental students. *Journal of the American Dental Association, 98*, 196–201.

Rutzen, S.R. (1973). The social importance of orthodontic rehabilitation: Report of a five year follow-up study. *Journal of Health and Social Behavior, 14*, 233–240.

Salter, A. (1949). *Conditioned reflex therapy: The direct approach to the reconstruction of personality*. New York: Creative Age Press.

Samelson, F. (1980). J.B. Watson's Little Albert, Cyril Burt's twins, and the need for a critical science. *American Psychologist, 35*, 619–625.

Sandler, J., & Dare, C. (1970). The psychoanalytic concept of orality. *Journal of Psychosomatic Research, 14*, 211–222.

Sarnat, H., Peri, J.N., Nitzan, E., & Perlberg, A. (1972). Factors which influence cooperation between dentist and child. *Journal of Dental Education, 36*, 9–15.

Schachter, S., & Singer, J.E. (1962). Cognitive, social, and physiological determinants of emotional state. *Psychological Review, 69*, 379–399.

Schachter, S., & Wheeler, L. (1962). Epinephrine, chlorpromazine and amusement. *Journal of Abnormal and Social Psychology, 65,* 121–128.

Scher, J.M. (Ed.). (1962). *Theories of the mind.* New York: The Free Press of Glencoe.

Schuurs, A.H.B., Duivenvoorden, H.J., van Velzen, S.K.T., & Verhage, F. (1986). Fear of dental procedures. *Community Dental Health, 3,* 227–237.

Schwartz, R.A., Greene, C.S., & Laskin, D.M. (1979). Personality characteristics of patients with myofascial pain-dysfunction (MPD) syndrome unresponsive to conventional therapy. *Journal of Dental Research, 58,* 1435–1439.

Scott, D.S., & Hirschman, R. (1982). Psychological aspects of dental anxiety in adults. *Journal of the American Dental Association, 104,* 27–31.

Secord, P.F., & Backman, C.W. (1964). *Social psychology.* New York: McGraw-Hill.

Seligman, M.E.P. (1970). On the generality of the laws of learning. *Psychological Review, 77,* 406–418.

Seligman, M.E.P. (1971). Phobias and preparedness. *Behaviour Therapy, 2,* 307–321.

Seligman, M.E.P., & Hager, J.L. (Eds.) (1972). *Biological boundaries of learning.* New York: Appleton-Century-Crofts.

Selltiz, C., Jahoda, M., Deutsch, M., & Cook, S.W. (1963). *Research methods in social relations. Revised one-volume edition.* New York: Holt, Rinehart and Winston.

Shaw, L., Maclaurin, E.T., & Foster, T.D. (1986). Dental study of handicapped children attending special schools in Birmingham, UK. *Community Dentistry and Oral Epidemiology, 14,* 24–27.

Shoben, E.J., & Borland, L. (1954). An empirical study of the etiology of dental fears. *Journal of Clinical Psychology, 10,* 171–174.

Skevington, S.M. (1986). Psychological aspects of pain in rheumatoid arthritis: A review. *Social Science and Medicine, 23,* 567–575.

Skinner, B.F. (1953). *Science and human behavior.* New York: Macmillan.

Sommer, R. (1969). *Personal space: The behavioral basis of design.* Englewood Cliffs, N.J.: Prentice-Hall.

Speake, J.D. (1980). Caries prevalence and restorative dental services in some Pacific Islands. *Australian Dental Journal, 25,* 193–196.

Sternbach, R.A. (1968). *Pain: A psychophysiological analysis.* New York: Academic Press.

Sternbach, R.A. (1974). *Pain patients: traits and treatment.* New York: Academic Press.

Stokes, T.F., & Kennedy, S.H. (1980). Reducing child uncooperative behavior during dental treatment through modeling and reinforcement. *Journal of Applied Behavior Analysis, 13,* 41–49.

Strevel, D.W. (1982). Consumer choice between dental delivery systems. *Journal of the American Dental Association, 104,* 157–163.

Sutton, S.R. (1982). Fear-arousing communications: A critical examination of theory and research. In J.R. Eiser (Ed.), *Social psychology and behavioral medicine.* Chichester: Wiley.

Swain, J.J., Allard, G.B., & Holborn, S.W. (1982). The good toothbrushing game: A school-based dental hygiene program for increasing the toothbrushing effectiveness of children. *Journal of Applied Behavior Analysis, 15,* 171–176.

Sword, R.O. (1970). Oral neglect—why? *Journal of the American Dental Association, 80,* 1327–1330.

Szasz, T.S. (1968). The psychology of persistent pain: A portrait of l'homme douloureux. In A. Soulairac, J. Cahn, & J. Charpentier (Eds.) *Pain.* London: Academic Press.

Tajfel, H. (1981). *Human groups and social categories*. Cambridge: Cambridge University Press.

Tarachow, S. (1946). The relationship of the dentist to neurotic psychological types. *New York Journal of Dentistry, 16*, 189–195.

Taylor, J.A. (1953). A personality scale of manifest anxiety. *Journal of Abnormal and Social Psychology, 48*, 285–290.

Thorndike, E.L. (1932). *The fundamentals of learning*. New York: Teachers College.

Todes, C.J. (1972). The child and the dentist: A psychoanalytic view. *British Journal of Medical Psychology, 45*, 45–55.

Tursky, B. (1974). Physical, physiological, and psychological factors that affect pain reaction to electric shock. *Psychophysiology, 11*, 95–112.

Tursky, B. (1976). The development of a pain perception profile: A psychophysical approach. In M. Weisenberg & B. Tursky (Eds.), *Pain: New perspectives in therapy and research*. New York: Plenum.

Underwood, B.J. (1957). *Psychological research*. New York: Appleton-Century-Crofts.

Van Groenestijn, M.A.J., Maas-de Waal, C.J., Mileman, P.A., & Swallow, J.N. (1980a). The ideal dentist. *Social Science and Medicine, 14A*, 533–540.

Van Groenestijn, M.A.J., Maas-de Waal, C.J., Mileman, P.A., & Swallow, J.N. (1980b). The image of the dentist. *Social Science and Medicine, 14A*, 541–546.

Venham, L.L. (1979). The effect of mother's presence on child's response to dental treatment. *Journal of Dentistry for Children, 46*, 51–57.

Venham, L.L., Bengston, D., & Cipes, M. (1977). Children's response to sequential dental visits. *Journal of Dental Research, 56*, 454–459.

Venham, L.L., Bengston, D., & Cipes, M. (1978). Parent's presence and the child's response to dental stress. *Journal of Dentistry for Children, 45*, 213–217.

Venham, L.L., Murray, P., & Gaulin-Kremer, E. (1979a). Child-rearing variables affecting the preschool child's response to dental stress. *Journal of Dental Research, 58*, 2042–2045.

Venham, L.L., Murray, P., & Gaulin-Kremer, E. (1979b). Personality factors affecting the preschool child's response to dental stress. *Journal of Dental Research, 58*, 2046–2051.

Walsh, J.P. (1953). Psychogenic symptoms in dental practice. *Oral Surgery, Oral Medicine, and Oral Pathology, 6*, 437–443.

Walsh, J.P. (1956). The dentist-patient relationship. *Australian Dental Journal, 1*, 102–111.

Walsh, J.P. (1959). Diagnosis and treatment of some psychogenic disorders of dental interest. *New Zealand Dental Journal, 55*, 14–19.

Walsh, J.P. (1962). Psychostomatology. *New Zealand Dental Journal, 58*, 13–21.

Walsh, J.P. (1964). Psychological defence mechanisms in dentistry. *Australian Dental Journal, 9*, 455–465.

Walsh, J.P. (1965). The psychogenesis of Bruxism. *Journal of Periodontology, 36*, 417–420.

Wardle, J. (1982). Fear of dentistry. *British Journal of Medical Psychology, 55*, 119–126.

Wardle, J. (1983). Psychological management of anxiety and pain during dental treatment. *Journal of Psychosomatic Research, 27*, 399–402.

Wardle, J. (1984). Dental pessimism: Negative cognitions in fearful dental patients. *Behaviour Research and Therapy, 22*, 553–556.

Watson, J.B., & Rayner, R. (1920). Conditioned emotional reactions. *Journal of Experimental Psychology, 3*, 1–14.

Watson, J.F., Brundo, G.C., & Grenfell, J. (1979). Attitudinal differences of faculty and students regarding the care of special (handicapped) patients in a dental school clinic. *Journal of the American Dental Association, 98*, 395–397.

Weinstein, P., Getz, T., Ratener, P., & Domoto, P. (1982a). The effect of dentists' behaviors on fear-related behaviors in children. *Journal of the American Dental Association, 104*, 32–38.

Weinstein, P., Getz, T., Ratener, P., & Domoto, P. (1982b). Dentists' responses to fear- and nonfear-related behaviors in children. *Journal of the American Dental Association, 104*, 38–40.

Weinstein, P., Milgrom, P., Ratener, P., Read, W., & Morrison, K. (1978). Dentists' perceptions of their patients: Relation to quality of care. *Journal of Public Health Dentistry, 38*, 10–21.

Weinstein, P., Smith, T.A., & Bartlett, R.C. (1971). A study of the dental student-patient relationship. *Journal of Dental Research, 52*, 1287–1292.

Weisenberg, M. (1973). Behavioral motivation. *Journal of Periodontology, 44*, 489–499.

Weisenberg, M. (1980). Understanding pain phenomena. In S. Rachman (Ed.), *Contributions to medical psychology. Volume 2.* Oxford: Pergamon.

Weisenberg, M., & Epstein, D. (1973). Patient training as an alternative to general anesthesia. *New York State Dental Journal, 39*, 610–613.

Weisenberg, M., Kegeles, S.S., & Lund, A.K. (1980). Children's health beliefs and acceptance of a dental preventive activity. *Journal of Health and Social Behavior, 21*, 59–74.

White, M.V., Betz, N.E., & Beck, F.M. (1982). Dental patients' perceptions of women dentists. *Journal of the American Dental Association, 105*, 223–226.

White, W.C., Akers, J., Green, J., & Yates, D. (1974). Use of imitation in the treatment of dental phobia in early childhood: A preliminary report. *Journal of Dentistry for Children, 41*, 26–30.

Wicker, A.W. (1969). Attitudes versus actions: The relationship of verbal and behavioral responses to attitude objects. *Journal of Social Issues, 25*(4), 41–78.

Willard, D.H., & Nowak, A.J. (1981). Communicating with the family of the child with a developmental disability. *Journal of the American Dental Association, 102*, 647–650.

Winer, G.A. (1982). A review and analysis of children's fearful behavior in dental settings. *Child Development, 53*, 1111–1133.

Winkler, J.D., & Taylor, S.E. (1979). Preference, expectations, and attributional bias: Two field studies. *Journal of Applied Social Psychology, 9*, 183–197.

Wolpe, J. (1969). *The practice of behavior therapy.* New York: Pergamon.

Wolpe, J. (1981). Behavior therapy versus psychoanalysis: Therapeutic and social implications. *American Psychologist, 36*, 159–164.

Woodworth, R.S. (1959). *Contemporary schools of psychology.* London: Methuen.

Wozniczka, L.P. (1977). Illness-labelling: The application of social psychology to illness. B.Sc. (Honours) thesis, School of Psychology, University of New South Wales, Sydney, Australia.

Wright, F.A.C., & Lange, D.E. (1976). Dental anxiety and children. *New Zealand Dental Journal, 72*, 80–83.

Wright, G.Z., Alpern, G.D., & Leake, J.L. (1973a). A cross-validation of variables affecting children's cooperative behaviour. *Journal of the Canadian Dental Association, 39*, 268–273.

Wright, G.Z., Alpern, G.D., & Leake, J.L. (1973b). The modifiability of maternal anxiety as it relates to children's cooperative dental behavior. *Journal of Dentistry for Children, 40,* 265–271.

Wroblewski, P.F., Jacob, T., & Rehm, L.P. (1977). The contribution of relaxation to symbolic modeling in the modification of dental fears. *Behavior Research and Therapy, 15,* 113–115.

Yates, A.J. (1958). Symptoms and symptom substitution. *Psychological Review, 65,* 371–374.

Yates, A.J. (1975). *Theory and practice in behavior therapy.* New York: Wiley.

Yule, A.J. (1975). Dental health on Mornington Island. *Australian Dental Journal, 20,* 167–169.

Zborowski, M. (1969). *People in pain.* San Francisco: Jossey-Bass.

Zimbardo, P.G. (1969). The human choice: Individuation, reason, and order versus deindividuation, impulse, and chaos. In W.J. Arnold & D. Levine (Eds.), *Nebraska symposium on motivation, 17,* 237–307.

Author Index

Subject Index